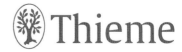

Imaging of Cerebrovascular Disease
A Practical Guide

Val M. Runge, MD
Editor-in-Chief of *Investigative Radiology*
Institute for Diagnostic, Interventional, and Pediatric Radiology
Inselspital, University Hospital of Bern
Bern, Switzerland

Thieme
New York • Stuttgart • Delhi • Rio de Janeiro

Executive Editor: William Lamsback
Managing Editor: J. Owen Zurhellen IV
Editorial Assistant: Mary B. Wilson
Director, Editorial Services: Mary Jo Casey
Production Editor: Heidi Grauel
International Production Director: Andreas Schabert
Vice President, Editorial and E-Product
    Development: Vera Spillner
International Marketing Director: Fiona Henderson
International Sales Director: Louisa Turrell
Director of Sales, North America: Mike Roseman
Senior Vice President and Chief Operating
    Officer: Sarah Vanderbilt
President: Brian D. Scanlan
Printer: Asia Pacific Offset

Library of Congress Cataloging-in-Publication Data

Runge, Val M., author.
Images of cerebrovascular disease : a practical guide /
Val M. Runge.
First edition. | New York : Thieme, [2016] | Includes
index.
LCCN 2015043822 (print) | LCCN 2015044294
    (ebook) | ISBN 9781626232488 (pbk.) | ISBN
    9781626232495 (e-ISBN) | ISBN 9781626232495
    (E-book)
MESH: Cerebrovascular Disorders—diagnosis—Atlases.
    | Cerebrovascular Disorders—pathology—Atlases. |
    Neuroimaging—methods—Atlases.
LCC RC388.5 (print) | LCC RC388.5 (ebook) | NLM WL
    17 | DDC 616.8/107543—dc23
LC record available at http://lccn.loc.gov/2015043822

Important note: Medicine is an ever-changing science undergoing continual development. Research and clinical experience are continually expanding our knowledge, in particular our knowledge of proper treatment and drug therapy. Insofar as this book mentions any dosage or application, readers may rest assured that the authors, editors, and publishers have made every effort to ensure that such references are in accordance with **the state of knowledge at the time of production of the book**.

Nevertheless, this does not involve, imply, or express any guarantee or responsibility on the part of the publishers in respect to any dosage instructions and forms of applications stated in the book. **Every user is requested to examine carefully** the manufacturers' leaflets accompanying each drug and to check, if necessary in consultation with a physician or specialist, whether the dosage schedules mentioned therein or the contraindications stated by the manufacturers differ from the statements made in the present book. Such examination is particularly important with drugs that are either rarely used or have been newly released on the market. Every dosage schedule or every form of application used is entirely at the user's own risk and responsibility. The authors and publishers request every user to report to the publishers any discrepancies or inaccuracies noticed. If errors in this work are found after publication, errata will be posted at www.thieme.com on the product description page.

Some of the product names, patents, and registered designs referred to in this book are in fact registered trademarks or proprietary names even though specific reference to this fact is not always made in the text. Therefore, the appearance of a name without designation as proprietary is not to be construed as a representation by the publisher that it is in the public domain.

Copyright © 2017 by Thieme Medical Publishers, Inc.

Thieme Publishers New York
333 Seventh Avenue, New York, NY 10001 USA
1 800 782 3488, customerservice@thieme.com

Thieme Publishers Stuttgart
Rüdigerstrasse 14, 70469 Stuttgart, Germany
+49 [0]711 8931 421, customerservice@thieme.de

Thieme Publishers Delhi
A-12, Second Floor, Sector-2, Noida-201301
Uttar Pradesh, India
+91 120 45 566 00, customerservice@thieme.in

Thieme Publishers Rio de Janeiro, Thieme Publicações Ltda.
Edifício Rodolpho de Paoli, 25º andar
Av. Nilo Peçanha, 50 – Sala 2508
Rio de Janeiro 20020-906 Brasil
+55 21 3172 2297

Cover design: Thieme Publishing Group
Typesetting by: Grauel Group
Printed in China by Asia Pacific Offset   5 4 3 2 1

ISBN 978-1-62623-248-8

Also available as an e-book:
eISBN 978-1-62623-249-5

With special thanks to Johannes Heverhagen, Juerg Hodler, Anton Valavanis, and the members of their departments at the University Hospitals of Bern and Zürich, Switzerland.

Contents

Foreword *by William G. Bradley Jr.* ix

Preface xi

Acknowledgments xii

Abbreviations xiii

Contributors xiv

Chapter 1	**Technologic Innovations in MR and CT** 1	
	Introduction 1	
	Magnetic Resonance (MR) 1	
	Computed Tomography (CT) 20	
	Summary 26	
Chapter 2	**Normal Anatomy** 27	
	Brain Parenchyma 27	
	Arterial Anatomy 29	
	Venous Anatomy 34	
	Common Anatomic Variants 37	
Chapter 3	**Hemorrhage** 39	
	Parenchymal Hemorrhage 39	
	Subarachnoid Hemorrhage 41	
	Superficial Siderosis 44	
Chapter 4	**Ischemia** 47	
	Introduction 47	
	Acute Cerebral Ischemia 48	
	Subacute Cerebral Infarcts 54	
	Chronic Cerebral Infarcts 60	
	Arterial Territory Infarcts 63	
	Watershed Infarcts 64	
	Multiple Embolic Infarcts 71	
	Lacunar Infarcts 72	
	Brainstem Infarcts 76	
	Gyral Localization of Cortical Infarcts 76	
	Small Vessel Ischemic Disease 83	
	Venous Infarcts 85	
	Less Common Presentations 88	
	Other Disease Entities That Feature or Mimic Ischemia 88	

Chapter 5 **Aneurysms** **95**
    Introduction. 95
    Aneurysm Treatment 98
    Intracranial Aneurysms by Location 103
    Subarachnoid Hemorrhage 110
    Other Aneurysm Subtypes. 117

Chapter 6 **Vascular Malformations and Other Vascular Lesions** **121**
    Arteriovenous Malformation 121
    Dural Arteriovenous Fistula. 125
    Carotid-Cavernous Fistula 129
    Cerebral Cavernous Malformation. 130
    Developmental Venous Anomaly. 133
    Capillary Telangiectasia 135
    Vertebrobasilar Dolichoectasia. 135
    Venous Thrombosis 136
    Vascular Lesions (Neck) 137

Index **141**

Foreword

In this pithy book, Dr. Val M. Runge has focused on imaging of cerebrovascular disease using MRI, CT, and DSA. This nicely complements two of his 16 previous books, *The Physics of Clinical MR Taught Through Images* and *Essentials of Clinical MR.* By focusing on cerebrovascular disease, he is able to go into greater depth than in any of his previous textbooks. As with his previous books, this tome is very image-rich and loaded with the latest information. For example, in Chapter 5, Aneurysms, he talks about treatment with surgery (clipping) and by endovascular techniques (e.g., coiling and flow diversion). He honestly points out the advantages and disadvantages of these techniques in terms of mortality and morbidity.

While this book has quite a bit of information, Dr. Runge's easy writing style makes it ideal for radiology, neurosurgery, and neurology residents and fellows. One might go so far to say it should be required reading for anyone dealing regularly with imaging of cerebrovascular disease or preparing to take Boards or CAQs. While clearly useful for trainees, it would also be useful for attending neuroradiologists, neurologists, and neurosurgeons. Personally I picked up quite a few tidbits when I read it. I hope you will enjoy it as much as I did.

William G. Bradley Jr., MD, PhD, FACR
Professor and Chair
Department of Radiology
University of California San Diego
San Diego, California

Preface

Imaging of Cerebrovascular Disease: A Practical Guide is written both to be read from cover to cover and to be used as a quick reference in the midst of a busy clinical day. It serves well as a supplement to general introductory neuroradiology texts, advancing the reader's expertise regarding ischemia, aneurysms, vascular malformations, and other vascular lesions. The text can also be used as a supplement for study prior to relevant certification exams, for example the American Board of Radiology Neuroradiology subspecialty exam. Designed as a practical educational resource for the imaging of cerebrovascular disease, it is divided into six chapters. The breadth of coverage is unparalleled, in terms of illustration with modern imaging techniques of the spectrum of ischemic lesions, as well as that of aneurysms and arteriovascular malformations, both prior to and following treatment. Attention is paid to detailed gyral anatomy in the chapter concerning brain ischemia, an important subtopic. Care has also been taken for the text to be inclusive, yet focusing on the most important disease presentations, covering well the breadth of the topic without gaps.

The diseases and their imaging presentations that are likely to be encountered in clinical practice and that are essential to know are covered comprehensively. The focus is on illustrating and describing the relevant findings as visualized on MR, CT, and digital subtraction angiography (DSA), as well as providing in-depth discussion. The text is written from a clinical imaging perspective, drawing on both personal experience and traditional education resources. In this way, it also covers common imaging findings often not well described in more traditional, multi-author, academic textbooks. The true basis of the text is that of the clinical imaging of cerebrovascular disease and recognition of characteristic findings on MR, CT, and DSA of the disease processes we are likely to encounter in clinical practice, using as a basis excellent images and case material from all three modalities.

Acknowledgments

Portions of my previous books entitled *Clinical 3T Magnetic Resonance* (Thieme 2007), *The Physics of Clinical MR Taught Through Images, 3rd Edition* (Thieme 2014), and *Neuroradiology: The Essentials with MR and CT* (Thieme 2015) were incorporated with permission in the current text. Portions of the articles entitled "Technological Advances in CT, and the Clinical Impact Therein" (Runge VM et al) and "MRI and CT of the Brain, 50 Years of Innovation, With a Focus on the Future" (Runge VM et al), published in *Investigative Radiology* (*Invest Radiol* 2015;50(2):119–127 and 2015;50[9]), respectively, have also been used with permission.

Abbreviations

The following abbreviations are used with the figures to enable rapid recognition of imaging technique and to permit the legends to be more concise.

ADC	apparent diffusion coefficient
ASL	arterial spin labeling
CBF	cerebral blood flow
CBV	cerebral blood volume
CE CT	contrast enhanced CT
CE MRA	contrast enhanced magnetic resonance angiography
CE PC	contrast enhanced phase contrast angiography
CE T1	contrast enhanced T1-weighted
CE T1 FS	contrast enhanced T1-weighted, with fat suppression
CT	computed tomography
CTA	CT angiography
DSA	digital subtraction angiography
DWI	diffusion weighted imaging
FLAIR	fluid attenuated inversion recovery
FSE (TSE)	fast spin echo (turbo spin echo)
GRE	gradient recalled echo, specifically with T2* weighting
MTT	mean transit time
PC	phase contrast angiography
PD	proton density weighted
PET	positron emission tomography
SI	signal intensity
STIR	short tau inversion recovery
SWI	susceptibility weighted imaging
T1	T1-weighted
T1 FS	T1-weighted, with fat suppression
T2	T2-weighted
T2 FS	T2-weighted, with fat suppression
TE	echo time
TOF	time of flight magnetic resonance angiography
TR	repetition time
CE TOF	contrast enhanced time of flight magnetic resonance angiography
TTP	time to peak
VRT	volume rendering technique

Contributors

Prof. dr. Wieslaw L. Nowinski, DSc, PhD
Founding Director
Center for Virtual Anatomy and Surgical
   Simulation
Cardinal Stefan Wyszynski University
Warsaw, Poland

Rüdiger von Ritschl, MD
Director of Neuroimaging
Superior Imaging
Windsor, Ontario, Canada

Val M. Runge, MD
Editor-in-Chief of *Investigative Radiology*
Institute for Diagnostic, Interventional, and
   Pediatric Radiology
Inselspital, University Hospital of Bern
Bern, Switzerland

1 Technologic Innovations in MR and CT

■ Introduction

Both CT and MR have made tremendous technologic advances since their clinical introduction, regarding not only sensitivity and spatial resolution, but also in terms of the speed of image acquisition. Advances in CT in recent years have focused in part on reduced radiation dose, an important topic for the years to come. MR has seen the development of a plethora of scan techniques, with marked superiority to CT in terms of tissue contrast due to the many parameters that can be assessed and their intrinsic sensitivity. Future advances in MR for clinical practice will likely focus both on new acquisition techniques that offer advances in speed and resolution, such as simultaneous multislice imaging and data sparsity, and on standardization and further automation of image acquisition and analysis. Functional imaging techniques including specifically perfusion will be further integrated into the workflow to provide pathophysiologic information that influences differential diagnosis, to assist treatment decision and planning, and to identify and follow treatment-related changes.

■ Magnetic Resonance (MR)

Three-tesla MR imaging represents one of the major forefronts of diagnostic neuroradiology today, with 3 T currently considered the field strength of choice for brain imaging. Little more than a decade ago, information regarding routine clinical application was generally lacking due to rapid changes in instrumentation and the relatively small installed base; however, today 3 T is mature as a modality for clinical evaluation of the brain. Despite this statement, further substantial progress in terms of refining and improving technique

is anticipated in the years to come. Particularly because of research in the field of data sparsity, scan times for many applications are anticipated to decrease further in the future, in many instances substantially. 3 T offers higher signal-to-noise ratio (SNR) when compared to lower field strengths, an advantage that can be employed either for improved spatial resolution or to scan faster, the latter being important for in-patient imaging. This has led to a divergence of protocols, with longer high-resolution scans on one end and faster lower resolution scans on the other. A reduction in slice thickness for routine brain imaging is also an option with 3 T (both with 2D multislice imaging and 3D imaging). Today, 2D multislice scans of the brain are routinely acquired with a 4-mm slice thickness at 3 T, compared to 5 mm at 1.5 T. With 3D techniques, at 3 T, 1-mm sections are routinely acquired. It is quite likely that slice thickness for routine screening 2D brain exams will be further reduced in the future (for example, to 2 mm), with implementation of simultaneous multislice (slice accelerated) and/or data sparsity techniques—two active areas of research.

Brain imaging at 3 T, from a theoretical point of view, offers the potential for up to a factor of two increase in SNR when compared to 1.5 T, which would translate to a four-fold decrease in scan time if all other factors were held constant. However, since its clinical introduction, it has been clear that much of the increase in SNR would be used for improved spatial resolution. For neuroradiologists who have read large numbers of 1.5- and 3-T exams, it is readily evident that the higher quality of 3-T brain exams, due to higher spatial resolution and a mild decrease in scan time, equates to both markedly improved diagnostic quality and a scan that is easier and requires less time to interpret.

In the meantime, since its clinical introduction, a range of technical problems at 3 T have had to be overcome. These included accentuated motion artifacts (depending on imaging technique), heat deposition/specific absorption ratio (SAR) limits, and the prolongation of T1 with field strength.

Spatial Resolution

The improved SNR at 3 T leaves the neuroradiologist with a difficult decision, as illustrated in **Fig. 1.1**. High-resolution scans can be acquired with exquisite detail, or depending on the need and ability of the patient to

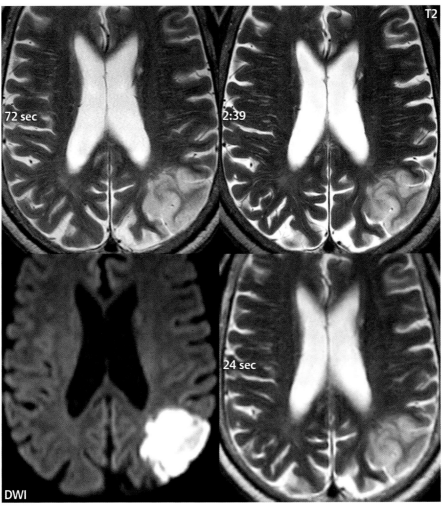

Fig. 1.1 Spatial resolution. MR images at 3 T are presented of a 69-year-old woman with a past medical history of hypertension, tobacco abuse, and multiple previous transient ischemic attacks (TIAs). She presented to the emergency department with right-sided weakness for 2 days and difficulty with speech. An early subacute infarct is noted, involving the posterior division of the left middle cerebral artery (MCA) and the adjacent watershed territory. The first image illustrates the screening T2-weighted scan that was employed at 3 T, using fast spin echo technique with 3-mm sections covering the entire brain, acquired in 72 seconds. A second T2-weighted acquisition is also shown, with higher in-plane spatial resolution (using the same slice thickness, 3 mm, as the initial scan), requiring a scan time of 2:39 min:sec. Both scans employed a parallel imaging factor of 2. On the diffusion weighted scan, the infarct demonstrates restricted diffusion (cytotoxic edema). The final T2-weighted scan presents one of many imaging approaches for noncooperative patients. This T2-weighted scan employed a parallel imaging factor of 3, reduced in-plane resolution, and a thicker slice section (5 mm) to achieve a scan time of 24 seconds using fast spin echo technique. Incidental to the case is a small chronic left caudate head lacunar infarct.

cooperate, very rapid scan sequences can be acquired. The current screening brain exam at 3 T, if performed with 2D technique, includes a 4-mm sagittal T1-weighted short TE gradient echo scan together with 4-mm axial fast spin echo (FSE) FLAIR and T2-weighted scans, and a 4-mm readout-segmented, multishot, axial diffusion-weighted scan, requiring a total scan time between 5 and 10 minutes. Sacrificing spatial resolution, such as imaging with 5-mm slices and/or using a lower in-plane resolution, scan times can be further reduced. Overall, the improved SNR at 3 T permits thinner sections to be acquired on a routine basis, combined with a modest reduction in scan time as compared with imaging at 1.5 T, decreasing motion artifacts as well as allowing improved imaging of uncooperative patients. This approach also allows rapid imaging when time is critical, such as in the diagnosis and management of acute stroke patients.

One caveat is important to mention in regard to in-plane spatial resolution. Although 3 T offers the ability to acquire an in-plane resolution in the brain well less than 0.5×0.5 mm^2, the consequences of this must be judged. Consider the use of T2-weighted FSE technique. Protocoling scans with variable in-plane (and through-plane) resolution, all with reasonable SNR, three possible options for example would be scans with voxel dimensions of $0.7 \times 0.7 \times 4$, $0.4 \times 0.4 \times 4$, and $0.4 \times 0.4 \times 2.5$ mm^3, with respective scan times of 30 sec, 1:30 min:sec, and 3:00 min:sec. However, stroke patients represent a subpopulation in which inadvertent motion is often a problem in regard to scan quality. To ask such a patient to hold still—meaning moving well less than one half of a millimeter—for a 3-minute scan with an in-plane resolution of $< 0.5 \times 0.5$ mm^2 and a slice thickness < 3 mm is simply not practical.

Slice Thickness

In this and subsequent sections, results at 1.5 and 3 T in the same patient will often be directly compared, acquired as part of an Institutional Review Board–approved study. The two MR units used in this comparison were located in adjacent clinical bays, allowing patients to be scanned easily at both field strengths in a single time slot. The MR systems (from Siemens Medical Solutions) were as closely matched as possible, with identical gradient coils and comparable head coils (identical geometry, design, and number of coils).

Slice thickness in MR has decreased steadily since its clinical introduction. In the early 1980s, 10 mm was the standard slice thickness for brain imaging. With time, as magnets were introduced using higher field strengths, slice thickness decreased to 7 mm (at 1.0 T) and then eventually to 5 mm. The latter represents the current standard for brain imaging at 1.5 T. With the improved SNR at 3 T, it is possible to further reduce the routine slice thickness used for brain imaging with preservation of image quality.

The SNRs for the four scans in **Fig. 1.2**, from region of interest measurements in white matter, were (1.5 T) 21 and (3 T) 63, 29, and 15 (only the upper left hand image was acquired at 1.5 T). As expected, there is a substantial improvement in SNR at 3 T, when slice thickness is held constant, with the 5 mm section at 1.5 T having an SNR of 21 and that at 3 T an SNR of 63. Theoretically, if all factors were held exactly constant, there should not be more than a two-fold improvement in SNR at 3 T. In the images shown, the SNR at 3 T is similar to that at 1.5 when using half the slice thickness (lower vs upper image, left side). However, as one can see in this case, the SNR of the 5-mm 1.5-T image actually falls in between that of the 2.5-mm and 1-mm images at 3 T. Looking at this from a strict visual perspective, the "graininess" of the 5-mm 1.5-T image is between that of the 2.5-mm and 1-mm sections at 3 T. The improvement beyond what is expected (a factor of 2 in SNR at 3 T) likely represented further hardware/software optimization on the 3-T system. In a real-world setting, the bandwidth of the 1.5-T acquisition would also have been increased (with matched pixel shift for the two field strengths), decreasing slightly the advantage of 3 T in terms of SNR.

As a further comment, imaging with thinner slices would not have been feasible without the advent of PACS and the filmless radiology department. The thinner slice thickness, which is very manageable in terms of clinical

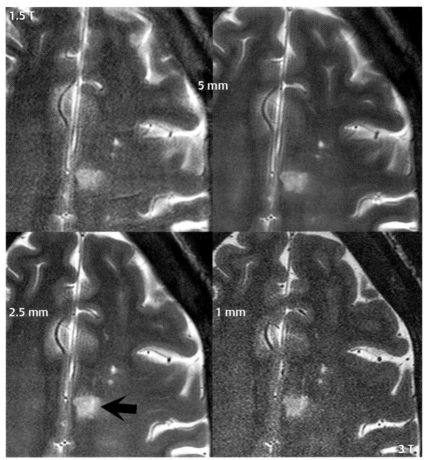

Fig. 1.2 Slice thickness. Illustrated is the improved SNR at 3 T and its implications in regard to slice thickness. The first scan was acquired at 1.5 T using a 5-mm slice thickness. This is compared with three subsequent 3 T scans, acquired with slice thicknesses of 5, 2.5, and 1 mm. The images are from a 36-year-old poorly controlled diabetic with known atherosclerotic vascular disease. They show a 1.5-cm area of vasogenic edema consistent with an early subacute segmental anterior cerebral artery infarction (*arrow*, 2.5-mm 3 T image). This region also demonstrated restricted diffusion (high SI on DWI, low ADC, image not shown). In addition, there are two tiny remote cavitated left frontal white matter infarcts. Fast spin echo (FSE) heavily T2-weighted images are illustrated with TR, TE, bandwidth, and number of echoes held constant. Scan time was also held constant, with each scan requiring 90 seconds for acquisition. Note that a substantially thinner slice, 2.5 mm, with improved diagnostic quality compared to 1.5 T, can be acquired at 3 T in the same scan time as the 5-mm-thick slice at the lower field strength. The 1-mm section at 3 T suffers from low SNR, although portions of the image appear sharper due to less through-plane partial volume imaging.

interpretation in the PACs environment, gives the reader a combination of improved image quality (less partial volume imaging), increased structural detail, and improved lesion detectability (for very small lesions).

It should be kept in mind when moving to thinner sections at 3 T that visualization of small punctate lesions will typically be improved. This is due to less partial volume imaging, with implications for scan interpretation when comparing exams from different field strengths. For example, with chronic small-vessel white ischemic disease, thinner sections can make the degree of involvement appear more prominent (with improved visualization of the areas of gliosis and with disease seen on more images due to the thinner sections).

Brain Screening

3 T offers unparalleled image quality for routine clinical brain MR, and specifically for brain ischemia. What follows is simply one possible protocol for brain screening at 3 T, implemented considering the trade-offs of scan time and image quality. Due to the large number of inpatients in our facility, the decision was made to keep scan times below 2 minutes for each scan sequence using 2D imaging with an in-plane resolution similar to that used at 1. 5 T, but with a 3-mm slice thickness as opposed to 5 mm at the lower field strength.

A 3-mm 2D short TE (2.4 msec) spoiled gradient echo sagittal T1-weighted scan is first acquired, with an acquisition time of 1:16 min:sec. This has excellent gray-white matter differentiation and thus also excellent visualization of vasogenic edema. Axial scans are subsequently acquired, all also with a 3-mm slice thickness, employing FSE T2-weighted and FLAIR scans, and diffusion weighted scans, with acquisition times of 1:32, 2:08, and 1:23 min:sec, respectively. The diffusion weighted scan in this approach is, however, a single shot technique, which has disadvantages in terms of bulk susceptibility artifacts, geometric distortion, and image blur (this topic is discussed in greater detail later on, and for a more in-depth consideration of MR physics, the reader is referred to *The Physics of Clinical MR Taught Through Images*, 3rd Edition [Thieme 2014]). Including the localizer, the entire acquisition time for this screening exam is 6:42 min:sec. This represents a reduction in scan time of 40% as compared to our routine exam at that time at 1.5 T, despite the reduction in slice thickness from 5 mm to 3 mm.

In regard to T1-weighted imaging of the brain, the use of a short in-phase TE (2.4 msec) 2D spoiled gradient echo (GRE) sequence is advocated. The short TE limits flow-related and susceptibility artifacts. This sequence is robust and does not experience significant specific absorption ratio limitations, poor tissue contrast, or accentuated motion artifacts as can be encountered with FSE or FLAIR T1-weighted imaging at 3 T. Comparing directly T1-weighted spin echo imaging at 1.5 T and the short TE GRE scan at 3 T (**Fig. 1.3**), the latter

offers superior SNR and contrast-to-noise ratio (CNR) with reduced motion artifacts and scan time. Use of this scan postcontrast is also critical to minimize pulsation artifacts from vascular structures. Thus, despite statements in the early literature to the contrary, excellent T1-weighted images of the brain can easily be acquired at 3 T by use of a short TE 2D GRE scan, a critical point for imaging of brain ischemia and the detection of methemoglobin (which is seen as high signal intensity on T1-weighted scans).

One important caveat to note, however, is that the appearance of arteries (and to a lesser extent veins) on both pre- and postcontrast scans is different with the short TE 2D GRE sequence at 3 T in comparison with the conventional T1-weighted FSE sequence typically employed at 1.5 T. On the GRE T1-weighted scan, precontrast, many of the larger proximal arteries are high signal intensity (as opposed to a flow void, seen with FSE technique), including specifically portions of the anterior (MCA) and posterior (basilar artery, PCA) circulations. Postcontrast on the GRE T1-weighted scan, there is relatively uniform enhancement of both intracranial arteries and veins, whereas with FSE technique, these are generally low signal intensity (a "flow void").

3 T also makes possible acquisition of diffusion weighted scans with substantially improved in-plane resolution, to be discussed in depth subsequently. An important further consideration, in terms of diffusion weighted imaging (DWI), is the implementation of a readout-segmented, multishot acquisition, also discussed subsequently, which markedly improves the bulk susceptibility artifacts otherwise seen at 3 T. A negative for this approach is that scan time is prolonged, in comparison to a single-shot echo planar DWI scan. However, an additional positive outcome is that image blur is markedly reduced.

Contrast Media

Contrast enhancement of brain lesions using the gadolinium chelates at 3 T is substantially improved when compared to 1.5 T (**Fig. 1.4**). Although the lower T1 relaxivity at higher

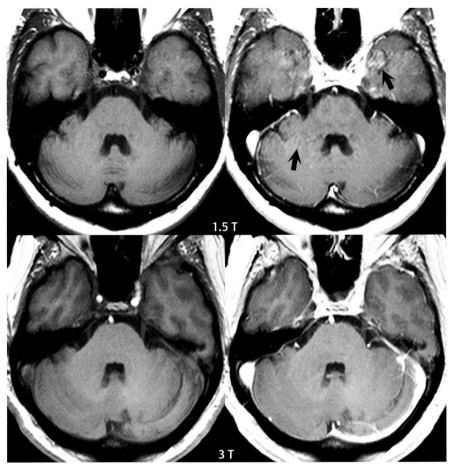

Fig. 1.3 2D short TE GRE T1-weighted imaging at 3 T. Illustrated is an age-matched comparison of pre- (left column) and postcontrast (right column) images acquired at 1.5 (upper row) with fast spin echo (FSE) and 3 T (lower row) with gradient recalled echo (GRE) technique. Scan times were 3:44 (pre) and 5:02 (post), for a 5-mm slice, at 1.5 T as compared to 1:11 (pre and post), for a 3-mm slice, at 3 T. Note the vascular pulsation artifacts on the 1.5-T study (arising from the internal carotid arteries anteriorly and the transverse sinuses posteriorly), accentuated postcontrast (*arrows*), despite the use of gradient moment nulling (flow compensation). No ghosting is evident on the 3-T study. The standard default 2D T1-weighted scan sequence at 1.5 T is FSE, whereas that at 3 T is a gradient echo (GRE). Thus the pulsation artifacts with the FSE scan are avoided (as they would be further accentuated at 3 T), with markedly diminished artifacts on the GRE scan due to the use of a short TE, typically close to 2.4 msec.

field strength for the gadolinium chelates (the intravenous agents used) would lead, in the absence of other factors, to lower enhancement, this is outweighed by the longer T1s that are intrinsic to 3 T in comparison to 1.5 T. The 2D short TE GRE T1-weighted scan is an excellent scan technique for postcontrast images and can be rapidly acquired in all three orthogonal planes (in 2 minutes or less for each scan). It is often implemented today with a slice thickness of 4 mm and a relatively high in-plane spatial resolution.

3D T1-weighted scans can also be used for postcontrast imaging, with two important caveats. If the same scan technique is not employed pre- and postcontrast, then it is possible to mistake a slightly hyperintense lesion (which appears that way due to the difference in scan technique) as one that enhances. Furthermore, MP-RAGE (also known by the terms 3D FGRE and 3D TFE) is commonly used at 3 T for postcontrast imaging, due to its appealing high gray-white matter contrast. However, as implemented, it is not that sensitive

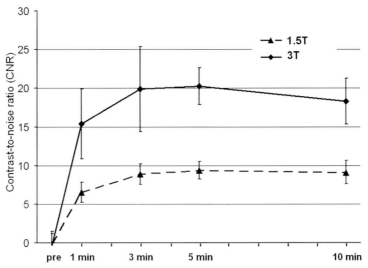

Fig. 1.4 Contrast enhancement. Lesion contrast-to-noise ratio (CNR), a quantitative measure of lesion enhancement, is depicted for different time points postcontrast, using an extracellular gadolinium chelate applied in a brain animal model at both 3 T and 1.5 T, with identical scan techniques. CNR at 3 T is consistently greater than that at 1.5 T for each time point, with the percent increase varying from 101 to 137%. Clinical results at 3 T show somewhat less than this degree of increase. In the results presented, bandwidth was not adjusted for field strength, and spin echo as opposed to the short TE gradient echo technique was employed. Each factor by itself has a negative effect in the range of 20%.

a technique for contrast enhancement. Other less commonly employed T1-weighted scans, such as 3D SPACE (also known by the terms CUBE and VISTA), are well known for their improved detectability of contrast enhancement, which translates into improved detection of small or poorly enhancing lesions. This difference in sensitivity of the technique has been well shown for intracranial metastatic disease, with SPACE greatly outperforming MP-RAGE in published studies in which both scans were acquired, in random temporal sequence, holding scan time and voxel dimensions constant.

3D Time of Flight MRA

3 T represents a major step forward in image quality for time of flight (TOF) MR angiography (MRA). This is nowhere more evident than in 3D TOF MRA of the circle of Willis. The lengthening of T1 at 3 T is in part responsible for this marked improvement. TOF contrast is based on the visualization of fresh unsaturated blood, which has not yet reached steady state, flowing into the excitation volume. The rate at which the flow of blood approaches steady state is based on TR and flip angle, from a pulse sequence perspective, and T1 and flow characteristics from a physiological perspective. At 3 T, T1 prolongation (due to field strength) results in the steady state signal level for stationary tissue being reduced, providing greater vessel contrast. This lessens the need for the use of magnetization transfer, permitting the use of shorter TRs and lower flip angles to increase depth penetration.

The net result is improved visualization at 3 T of both large and small arteries, on the basis of higher acquired spatial resolution and sufficient SNR to permit this. Aneurysm depiction is markedly improved (**Fig. 1.5**). However, like at 1.5 T, when there is slow flow, such as the delayed filling seen in very large aneurysms, the entire patent portion of the abnormality may not be visualized on the TOF study. Vessel occlusions and stenoses, together with reduced vessel caliber and slower flow, are also well visualized at 3 T, with the improved spatial resolution and overall image quality making such findings often much

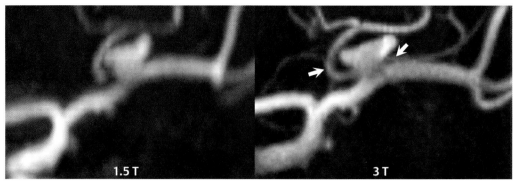

Fig. 1.5 3D time of flight MR angiography, a comparison of imaging at 1.5 and 3 T. Targeted MIP images of a multilobed 8-mm MCA aneurysm, arising from the M1 segment, are presented. In this case, the greater SNR and CNR available at 3 T have been used in part to improve spatial resolution. Two small branch vessels (*arrows*) originate from the aneurysm, a critical imaging finding, with the origin of the larger vessel not depicted and the smaller vessel itself not even evident on the 1.5 T scan. Voxel dimensions were $0.8 \times 0.8 \times 1$ mm^3 at 1.5 T and $0.4 \times 0.4 \times 0.4$ mm^3 at 3 T, with scan times of 6:08 and 8:28 min:sec, respectively.

more evident (**Fig. 1.6**, Parts 1 and 2). The excellent visualization of both small arteries and distal branching vessels intracranially, illustrated in figures throughout this text, is a consistent result with 3D TOF MRA at 3 T.

Diffusion Weighted Imaging

3 T offers for the first time the ability to do high in-plane resolution, as well as thin section diffusion weighted imaging (DWI), as illustrated in **Fig. 1.7** (Parts 1, 2, and 3). Shown are applications of DWI that have not been possible at 1.5 T. Thin section DWI has the same benefits as that of thin section T1- and T2-weighted imaging, described elsewhere, including improved anatomic detail and lesion detectability. High in-plane resolution diffusion weighted images also have not been clinically feasible at 1.5 T due to SNR limitations. These are routinely acquired at 3 T, albeit requiring a slightly longer scan time. Higher resolution DWI scans have substantially improved image detail compared to the 128×128 matrix scans acquired typically at 1.5 T (with 2×2 mm^2 in-plane resolution). Margins of the abnormalities are more distinct and smaller punctate areas of diffusion abnormality better seen. Utilizing thinner sections in combination with higher in-plane resolution diffusion weighted images, both easily performed at 3 T, leads to improved image quality and better detection of small infarcts, as illustrated in **Fig. 1.8** and later examples.

One negative feature of 3 T, at least in some applications, is the increase in bulk susceptibility artifact versus 1.5 T, since magnetic susceptibility scales linearly with field strength (**Fig. 1.9**, Parts 1 and 2). This is particularly evident in DWI. Parallel imaging plays an important role in improving DWI from this perspective, with each increment in parallel imaging factor decreasing the degree of artifact. It should be noted, however, that the degree of bulk susceptibility artifact from the air-filled sinuses, together with the degree of anatomic distortion, is quite variable from patient to patient at 3 T. The introduction of readout-segmented, multishot DWI has led to a further marked improvement in image quality and is today usually implemented at 3 T in combination with parallel imaging.

Artifacts arising from motion-induced phase errors pose a particular challenge in diffusion weighted imaging, leading to the use of single-shot echo planar imaging (ss-EPI) to overcome problems such as ghosting. However, the image quality of ss-EPI DWI suffers from relatively low spatial resolution, low SNR, and bulk susceptibility artifacts generated by tissue interfaces and metal implants. With increasing field strength, specifically

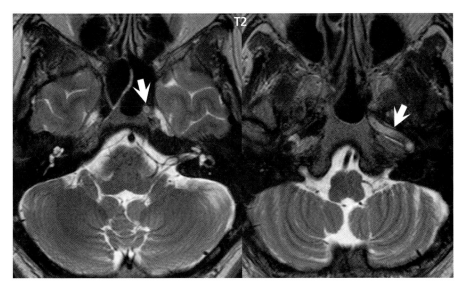

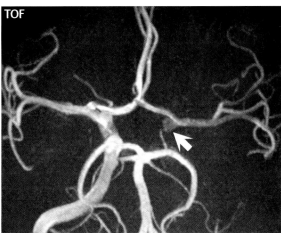

Fig. 1.6 Vessel occlusion and reduced arterial flow. All images were acquired at 3 T. (Part 1) T2-weighted axial images reveal abnormal high signal intensity within the petrous portion of the left internal carotid artery (*arrows*). This is consistent with either very slow flow or occlusion. (Part 2) An MIP projection of the 3D TOF MRA of the circle of Willis demonstrates occlusion of the petrous and cavernous portions of the left internal carotid artery, with only the carotid terminus (*arrow*) visualized. The left middle cerebral artery is supplied via collateral flow from the anterior and left posterior communicating arteries. Duplex ultrasound confirmed the absence of flow in the left internal carotid artery. Note the reduced signal intensity and caliber of the left middle cerebral artery and its branches, relative to the normal right side, due to reduced and delayed flow.

when moving from 1.5 to 3 T, susceptibility artifacts and degradation of spatial resolution become more pronounced. Susceptibility artifacts with ss-EPI can be attributed to the inherently long readout time resulting from acquisition of the entirety of k space for a given slice in a single shot (i.e., using a single RF excitation pulse). To overcome the limitations of ss-EPI, diffusion-weighted, multishot

EPI sequences (including specifically readout-segmented [rs] EPI, also termed RESOLVE) have been introduced that incorporate a phase correction to avoid artifacts caused by shot-to-shot, motion-induced phase errors. Sampling only a subset of k space at each excitation with rs-EPI leads to shorter readout times and reduces artifacts from bulk susceptibility relative to ss-EPI (**Fig. 1.10**).

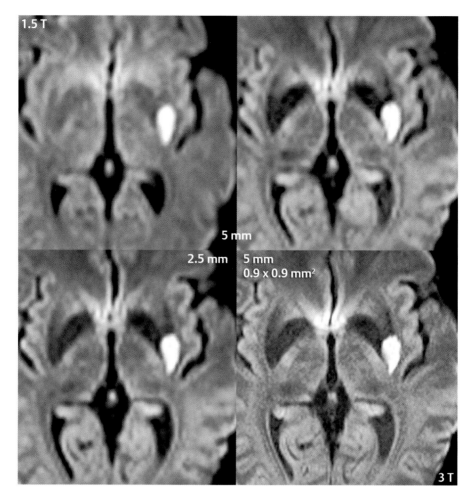

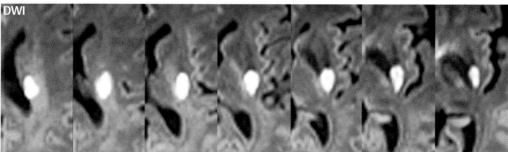

Fig. 1.7 Diffusion weighted imaging at 3 T, in comparison to 1.5 T. The images in Parts 1 and 2 are from a 57-year-old man with a history of hypertension who presented with right-sided facial droop together with right-sided upper and lower extremity weakness. An early subacute infarct is noted involving the left posterior periventricular white matter extending to involve the adjacent lentiform nucleus. The left uppermost image in Part 1 and the left hand image in Part 3 were obtained at 1.5 T (using a 5-mm slice thickness) with the remainder of the images acquired at 3 T. In Part 1, 5-mm and 2.5-mm-thick sections at 3 T are compared to the 5-mm section at 1.5 T. Also illustrated (lower right hand image) is a high in-plane spatial resolution diffusion weighted image acquired at 3 T using a 256 × 256 matrix (with an in-plane resolution of 0.9 × 0.9 mm² as compared to 1.9 × 1.9 mm² for the other scans). Part 2 illustrates 2.5-mm sections covering the craniocaudal extent of the infarct, thus showing the potential for thin section diffusion weighted imaging at 3 T. The images in Part 3 are from a 73-year-old man who presented to the emergency room with left arm weakness and unsteadiness. Early subacute infarcts are noted in the right MCA as well as right MCA/PCA watershed distributions. *(continued)*

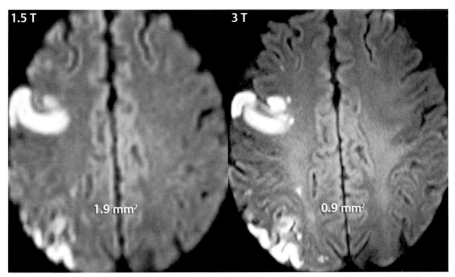

Fig. 1.7 *(Continued)* A 1.5-T image with conventional in-plane spatial resolution (for that field strength, 1.9 × 1.9 mm²) is compared to a 3-T image with substantially improved in-plane spatial resolution (0.9 × 0.9 mm²), the latter close in technique to that typically acquired in routine clinical practice at 3 T today.

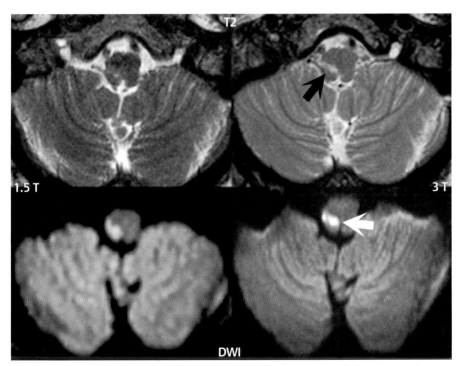

Fig. 1.8 Improved detection of a small, but clinically critical, infarct at 3 T. The images are from a 54-year-old diabetic with a 1-day history of ataxia. A small, early subacute right lateral medullary infarct is noted (*arrows*). Axial T2-weighted images are compared, with the slice thickness being 5 mm at 1.5 T and 3 mm at 3 T. Also compared are the respective diffusion weighted images, with that at 1.5 T being a 128 × 128 matrix, which is standard for this field strength, and that at 3 T being substantially higher resolution, specifically 256 × 256. This small medullary infarct is much better seen both on the thin section T2-weighted image at 3 T (*black arrow*) and on the high in-plane spatial resolution DWI at 3 T (*white arrow*).

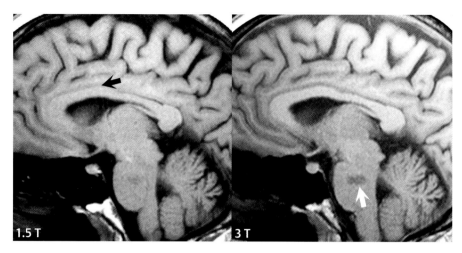

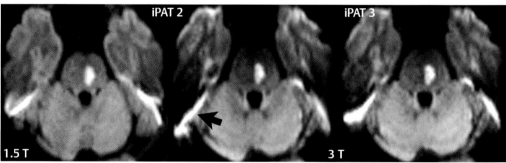

Fig. 1.9 Additional caveats to imaging technique at 1.5 and 3 T. The images in both Parts 1 and 2 are from a 57-year-old diabetic with a 1-day history of unsteadiness. (Part 1) Midline sagittal T1-weighted images depict an early subacute pontine infarct (*white arrow*) at 1.5 and 3 T. 2D spin echo technique was employed at 1.5 T with TR/TE = 550/12, a slice thickness of 5 mm, and a scan time of 2 min 55 sec. 2D gradient echo technique was employed at 3 T with TR/TE/tip angle = 440/2.4/90°, a parallel imaging factor of 2, a slice thickness of 3 mm, and a scan time of 1 min 15 sec. Gray-white matter contrast is similar between the two scans. The 1.5-T scan demonstrates a prominent ghost (*black arrow*), due to pulsation artifact from the superior sagittal sinus, with the 3-T scan artifact free. The improved depiction of the pontine infarct at 3 T is largely due to less partial volume imaging (3- vs 5-mm slice thickness).

(Part 2) An axial diffusion weighted image at 1.5 T (with a parallel imaging factor of 2 and three averages) is compared to two 3-T images for this same unilateral pontine infarct. The two 3-T scans had parallel imaging factors (iPAT) of 2 and 3, with the number of scan averages increased from two to three to compensate for the increase in iPAT. With the further increment in parallel imaging factor, the depiction of the pons, and specifically the left pontine infarct, is improved at 3 T. Note, however, that the bulk susceptibility artifact (when iPAT is held constant), seen in the region of the petrous apices bilaterally, is markedly worse at 3 T (*arrow*) as compared to 1.5 T. Image distortion, due to the sphenoid sinus and differences in susceptibility therein, is also greater at 3 T (for example, the pons is artificially "stretched" in the AP dimension), an effect that is less when iPAT is increased from 2 to 3.

Compared with ss-EPI, rs-EPI increases scan time due to the larger number of RF excitations (or shots) that are required to sample the k-space data required for each image. The end result is substantially improved image quality (**Fig. 1.11**) when ss-EPI (the primary approach at 1.5 T) is compared to rs-EPI (the recommended approach at 3 T), albeit with a longer scan time. The question of scan time leads further to the topic of simultaneous multislice (slice accelerated) diffusion EPI, discussed later.

Further Caveats (Edema, Motion, Hemorrhage)

Cytotoxic edema occurs within minutes of an ischemic event and is visualized on MR

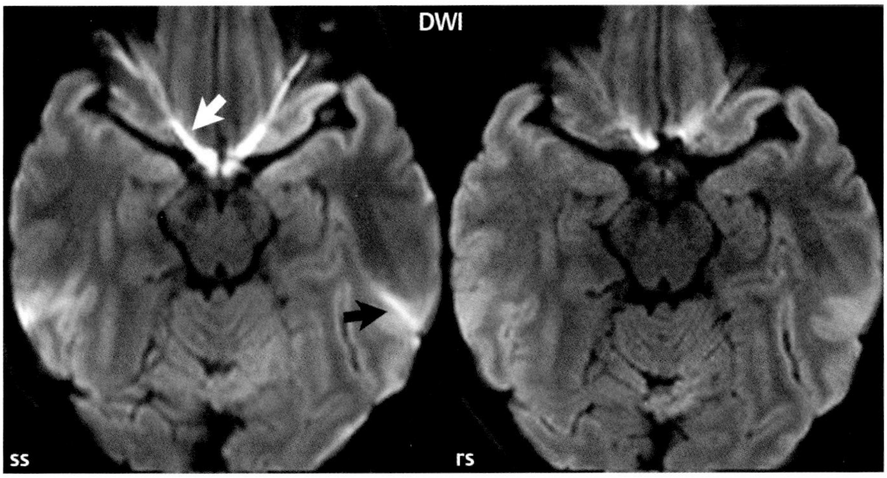

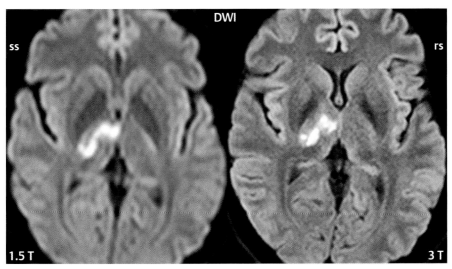

Fig. 1.10 Decreased bulk susceptibility artifact with implementation of readout-segmented (rs) echo planar imaging (EPI) for diffusion-weighted imaging. Representative images at 3 T compare a single-shot (ss) EPI sequence with an rs-EPI sequence (the latter also referred to by the term "multishot"), using the same parallel imaging factor and voxel size. Note both the decreased high signal intensity susceptibility artifact and the decreased artifactual blur with the rs-EPI. In the ss-EPI scan (formerly the standard sequence used for DWI), the artifact anteriorly (*white arrow*) is due to the sphenoid sinus and that posteriorly (*black arrow*) to the petrous apex and mastoid sinuses. The less extensive coverage of the frequency encoding dimension per shot in rs-EPI, when compared to ss-EPI (where all of k space is sampled with one excitation), enables the echo spacing to be decreased. The result is a decrease in both susceptibility artifacts and image blur. Regarding the latter, note the more sharply defined gray-white matter interface in the rs-EPI image, despite the same nominal in-plane resolution.

Fig. 1.11 Improved infarct depiction on DWI at 3 T in comparison to 1.5 T, employing rs-EPI. Scans at 1.5 and 3 T are illustrated in a patient with an early subacute right thalamic infarct, which also involves the posterior limb of the internal capsule. Note the marked improvement in image quality and lesion depiction when comparing 3 T to 1.5 T, the result of a higher pixel matrix in combination with the application of rs-EPI (as opposed to ss-EPI), with the SNR of 3 T making possible image acquisition using this technique in a reasonable scan time.

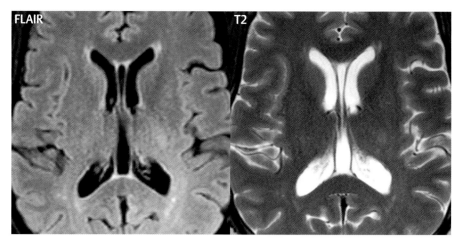

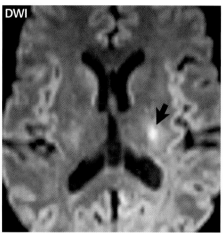

Fig. 1.12 The utility of diffusion weighted imaging for improved lesion detection. Presented are 3-mm axial (Part 1) FLAIR, FSE T2-weighted, and (Part 2) DWI images (with scan times of 1:30, 1:56, and 1:23 min:sec, respectively) from the 3-T scan of a 50-year-old male who presented to the emergency room with weakness involving the right half of the body, clumsiness, and slurred speech 12 hours prior to the MR exam. Abnormal high signal intensity (*arrow*) is seen on DWI near the interface between the lateral thalamus and posterior limb of the internal capsule on the left. The lesion was seen on three adjacent DWI slices, an advantage of thin section imaging, easing lesion recognition and diagnosis. On FLAIR and T2-weighted images, only a very subtle abnormal increase in signal intensity is visualized.

as restricted diffusion (high signal intensity on DWI). Vasogenic edema develops subsequently and is depicted on T2-weighted scans as abnormal high signal intensity. T2-weighted images are often normal within the first 8 hours following infarction, with the lesion becoming progressively hyperintense from 8 to 24 hours. Ninety percent of ischemic lesions will have abnormal high signal intensity on T2-weighted scans by 24 hours. The acute lacunar infarct illustrated in **Fig. 1.12** (Parts 1 and 2) demonstrates by MR a classic appearance, with predominantly cytotoxic edema and little if any vasogenic edema at this time point (12 hours). Differentiating between cytotoxic and vasogenic edema is important in cerebral ischemia, not only for determining the time frame of a lesion but also for prognostic and therapeutic considerations. In general, the lesion as seen on DWI is considered to represent the ischemic core, with the damage due to ischemia not reversible in this region.

Motion, regardless of origin, does in general cause greater artifacts at 3 T as opposed to 1.5 T. This includes arterial and venous pulsation artifacts and ghosts due to gross patient movement. Attention to details of scan technique can markedly reduce motion-related artifacts at 3 T. Advances in sequence design are also critical. Alternative scan techniques markedly reduce the impact of patient motion, with HASTE (for T2-weighted scans) and BLADE (for T2-weighted and FLAIR scans) both important in the imaging of cerebral ischemia. HASTE is robust in terms of motion artifacts due to the very rapid acquisition time (**Fig. 1.13**). However, edema is less

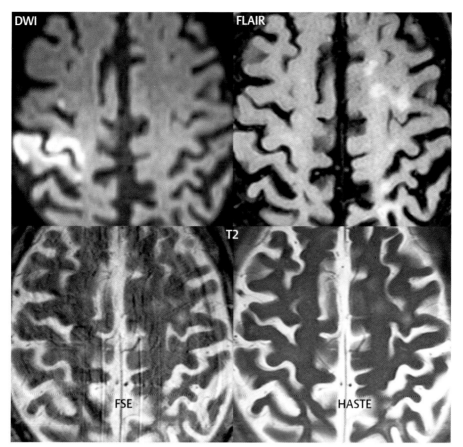

Fig. 1.13 Additional caveats for improved MR imaging of cerebral ischemia. Presented are 3-mm axial DWI, FLAIR, FSE, and HASTE T2-weighted images in an 80-year-old man with an acute (< 24 hours) infarct, all acquired at 3 T. Much like the imaging findings in Fig. 1.12, an abnormality is noted on DWI with little corresponding change on T2-weighted images. Abnormal high signal intensity is seen in the right pre- and postcentral gyri on DWI, reflecting cytotoxic edema. Little to no abnormality is noted in the corresponding location on T2-weighted scans (with vasogenic edema yet to develop). This case also illustrates the use at 3 T of HASTE, as an alternative to FSE T2-weighted imaging in uncooperative patients. Motion artifact in this instance substantially degrades the FSE T2-weighted scan. The acquisition time for this scan was 1:42 min:sec, with the scan being 2D multislice in type. The HASTE scan is acquired in single slice mode, with a scan time of 0.6 sec per slice, markedly limiting artifacts due to patient motion. Also noted on the scans in this individual is abnormal high signal intensity within the white matter of the centrum semiovale on the left, best seen on FLAIR, the residual of a chronic left MCA distribution infarct.

well depicted, due to intrinsic lower contrast. BLADE can be implemented for both T2-weighted and FLAIR scans and is very effective in reducing artifacts (**Fig. 1.14**); however, scan times are generally longer. Due to the radial nature of the BLADE (also termed PROPELLER and MultiVane) acquisition scheme, pulsation and motion artifacts are expressed in a more benign way (as opposed to a rectilinear acquisition of k space), and specific motion correction can also be implemented.

The reader is referred to *The Physics of Clini cal MR Taught Through Images,* 3rd Edition (Thieme, 2014), for a more in-depth explanation of both HASTE and BLADE.

The imaging characteristics of hemorrhage differ little at 3 T from those at 1.5 T, other than the improved sensitivity to blood products that exhibit principally $T2^*$ effects (deoxyhemoglobin and hemosiderin) (**Fig. 1.15**, Parts 1 and 2). The appearance of methemoglobin on T1-weighted scans, as high signal

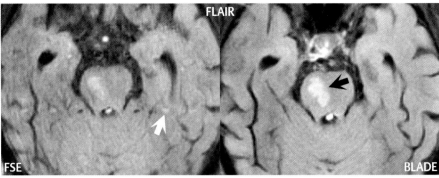

Fig. 1.14 The use of BLADE in uncooperative patients to reduce motion artifacts and improve image quality. Illustrated are FLAIR scans acquired with conventional (rectilinear k-space acquisition) FSE and BLADE. An acute pontine infarct (*black arrow*) is more clearly delineated in the BLADE scan, with the conventional scan degraded by gross motion artifacts and a prominent pulsation artifact (*white arrow*). If all other parameters are held constant, a BLADE scan will be 50% longer (which does have the beneficial effect of improved SNR), due to the inherent oversampling of the center of k space.

intensity, is unchanged (**Fig. 1.16**). Due to the greater T2* effects, both deoxyhemoglobin and hemosiderin will be more evident on scans acquired at 3 T, which can assist both in detection (for example of subarachnoid hemorrhage, petechial hemorrhage within an infarct, and small cavernous malformations) and in improved definition of involvement (**Fig. 1.17**, Parts 1 and 2). Unlike in DWI, where the greater sensitivity to susceptibility is responsible for larger artifacts at 3 T, in the detection of deoxyhemoglobin and hemosiderin, this is a distinct advantage of 3 T over lower field strengths.

Perfusion Imaging

Clinical perfusion techniques for MR employ tracers in two basic categories: diffusible (the tracer is not confined to the vessels and enters the tissue) and nondiffusible (the tracer is confined to the vessels). Arterial spin labeled (ASL) perfusion MRI is an example of a diffusible tracer technique. Arterial blood water is labeled and allowed to flow into the imaging plane(s), during which time there is T1 decay of the label. Multiple labeled/control image pairs are acquired and averaged. Subtraction of labeled images from unlabeled control images yields a difference image (**Fig. 1.18**), in which the signal change is proportional to cerebral blood flow (CBF).

Dynamic susceptibility contrast (DSC) MR is a nondiffusible perfusion technique. This approach involves analysis of the transient decrease in signal intensity on T2*-weighted images, observed during the first pass of contrast following intravenous bolus gadolinium chelate administration.

A limitation of ASL methods compared to DSC perfusion MR methods is low SNR. Signal changes in gray matter for DSC perfusion MR are on the order of 20 times higher than for ASL, explaining the use of a lower resolution acquisition matrix for ASL. Both ASL and DSC benefit from higher field strength, specifically 3 T. Another disadvantage to ASL, in addition to lower in-plane resolution, is the inability to obtain information regarding delayed transit, specifically mean transit time (MTT). However, an advantage to ASL, in comparison to DSC, is the ability to repeat the study (indeed multiple times) during a single patient exam. Regardless, DSC perfusion MR is by far the dominant technique in clinical practice today and is routinely acquired in patients presenting clinically with acute ischemia.

Dynamic susceptibility contrast perfusion imaging is performed by the acquisition of multiple, time sequential, single-shot echo planar imaging (EPI) slices measured with a temporal resolution of 1 sec or less during the bolus IV administration of a gadolinium chelate. The use of EPI enables rapid image acquisition with high sensitivity to the T2*

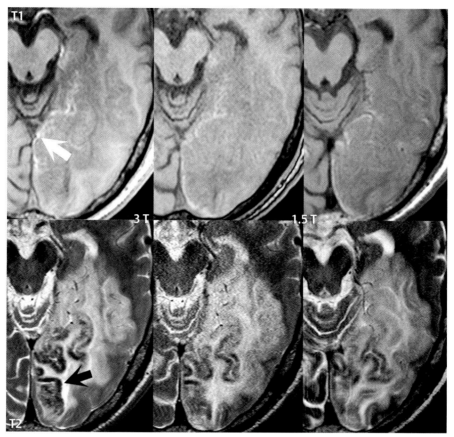

Fig. 1.15 Visualization of petechial hemorrhage in cerebral ischemia, focusing on T2* effects. The images are from the exam of an 83-year-old hypertensive man with atrial fibrillation who presented with a 1-week history of confusion and visual disturbances. (Part 1) There is a large, left, posterior cerebral artery, early subacute infarct, which demonstrates both petechial methemoglobin (*white arrow*) and deoxyhemoglobin (*black arrow*). On the top row, the left and middle images were acquired using the identical short TE 2D spoiled GRE sequence (with a slice thickness of 3 mm) but at 3 T as opposed to 1.5 T. The bandwidth, together with all other sequence parameters, was held constant. The graininess of the 1.5-T image reflects the lower SNR. The top row, right hand image is a routine 5-mm scan from 1.5 T, using spin echo technique. The scan times were 1:05, 1:05, and 4:49 min:sec, respectively. The bottom row presents a similar comparison for T2-weighted FSE imaging. The left and middle images were acquired using identical scan technique (with a slice thickness of 3 mm) but again at 3 T as opposed to 1.5 T. The difference in SNR between the images, with the 1.5-T image being low SNR and thus grainy in appearance, likewise primarily reflects the difference in field strength. The lower row, right hand image is a routine 5-mm T2-weighted scan from 1.5 T, using FSE technique and with the bandwidth optimized for 1.5 T. The scan times were 1:12, 1:12, and 1:29 min:sec, respectively. Note in both instances (T1- and T2-weighted scans) that the 3-mm 3-T images have similar to slightly improved SNR compared to the standard 5-mm scans at 1.5 T. (Part 2) Gradient echo T2*-weighted images are compared at 3 and 1.5 T in the same patient, again using identical imaging parameters. Note the markedly increased susceptibility effect at 3 T as compared to 1.5 T, and thus the improved visualization of deoxyhemoglobin (as gyriform low SI) in this subacute infarct. This effect can also be appreciated, albeit to a lesser extent, in comparing the FSE T2-weighted images at 3 and 1.5 T (Part 1). The graininess of the 1.5-T image in Part 2 reflects the markedly lower SNR at that field strength. (*continued*)

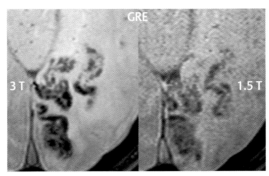

Fig. 1.15 (Continued)

effect of the contrast agent. Today's high-end MR scanners with advanced gradient technology are able to accommodate coverage of the entire brain with slices acquired in a dynamic fashion immediately prior to, during, and following passage of the contrast bolus through the brain. The transit of a gadolinium chelate (as a concentrated, compact bolus) through the brain causes a decrease in tissue signal intensity on echo planar images due to the T2* or magnetic susceptibility effect of the agent, with the temporal time curve observed. Using this acquired data, calculations are made to demonstrate the rate of change in the MR signal as well as the relative volume and flow of blood to the visualized area.

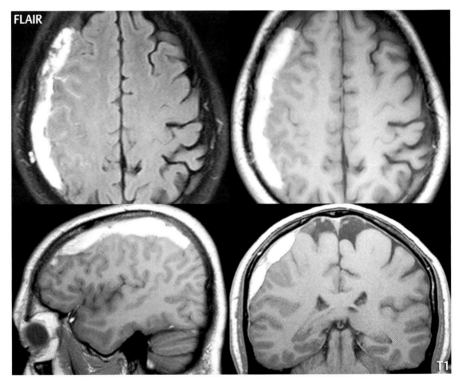

Fig. 1.16 Visualization of methemoglobin. Axial FLAIR and axial, sagittal, and coronal T1-weighted scans at 3 T in a young man with a subacute, extracellular methemoglobin subdural hematoma (high signal intensity on both T1- and T2-weighted scans). Note the exquisite depiction of the adjacent sulcal effacement. Methemoglobin appears as high signal intensity on T1-weighted scans, regardless of field strength.

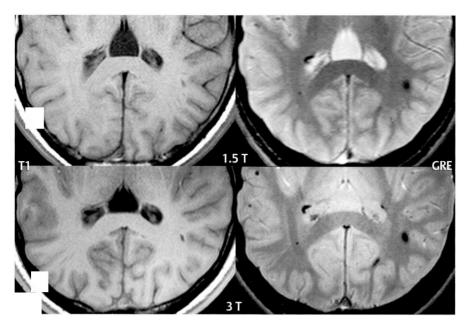

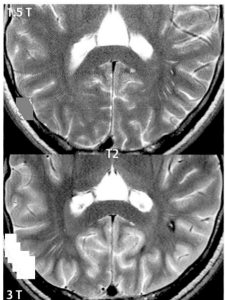

Fig. 1.17 Improved detection of small focal lesions at 3 T, on the basis of T2* effects. Scans are presented from a patient with multiple cavernous malformations, imaged at both 1.5 and 3 T. In Part 1, T1-weighted (left) and gradient echo T2*-weighted (right) scans are compared. In Part 2, T2-weighted fast spin echo scans are compared. The images at 1.5 T were 5 mm in slice thickness, as compared with 3 mm at 3 T. Scan times were comparable at 1.5 versus 3 T, with the exception that the T1-weighted scan required 3:09 (min:sec) at 1.5 T versus 1:05 at 3 T. Note the improved depiction of the many lesions in this patient at 3 T, in particular on the T2*-weighted image, due to a combination of the decreased slice thickness (reduced partial volume effect) together with the increased sensitivity to susceptibility effects. Examining each sequence pair (specifically the respective scans at 1.5 and 3 T), the lesions are best visualized at 3 T, with low signal intensity due to their hemosiderin content. The images at 1.5 T also appear slightly "grainy," due to poorer SNR.

Calculated results are displayed in the form of images or maps where each image is derived from the entire dynamic dataset for that slice position. The MTT map depicts the time required for fresh blood to completely replace that in the volume of interest. The cerebral blood volume (CBV) map conveys information regarding tissue blood volume within the displayed slice (**Fig. 1.19**). Note that normal gray and white matter are well differentiated on an CBV image due to the higher blood volume of gray matter. Cerebral blood flow (CBF) maps are also routinely calculated. These entities are related mathematically, specifically CBF = CBV/MTT. To obtain quantitative as opposed to relative values (for example, rCBV), measurement of the arterial input function is required.

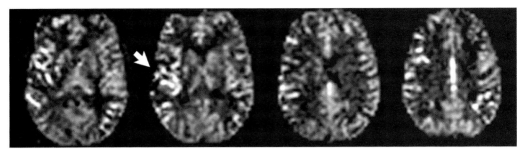

Fig. 1.18 Arterial spin labeling (ASL). Selected continuous ASL perfusion MR images from a patient with moyamoya syndrome are shown, acquired at 3 T. These demonstrate right greater than left high signal intensity in large vessels, predominantly in the right middle cerebral artery territory (*arrow*). The large vessel signal represents labeled spins experiencing enough of a delay that exchange with the microvasculature or tissue has not yet occurred. As with most scan techniques, ASL at 3 T is superior to that at 1.5 T, due to the inherent greater SNR.

Simultaneous Multislice (Slice Accelerated) Imaging

Simultaneous multislice (SMS) imaging employs an innovative acquisition and reconstruction scheme that allows multiple slices to be acquired simultaneously (the RF excitation is modified to excite multiple slices simultaneously), without a loss in SNR. The approach offers a substantial decrease in image acquisition time, or alternatively improved spatial/ diffusion resolution (including specifically the acquisition of thinner sections), depending on how it is applied. The advent of this technique is analogous to that of 2D multislice years ago and, as such, may represent one of the major innovations in this decade with widespread clinical utility. One result of combining readout-segmented EPI with slice acceleration is that a diffusion weighted scan can be acquired at 3 T with markedly reduced bulk susceptibility effect as well as image blur, with 2-mm slices through the entire brain, in a relatively short scan time (**Fig. 1.20**). The availability of simultaneous multislice imaging offers the possibility of implementing, for the imaging of brain ischemia, thinner sections (specifically, 2 mm) in routine clinical practice at 3 T (**Fig. 1.21**). SMS is currently available for both DWI and T2-weighted image sequences.

■ Computed Tomography (CT)

Current technologic advances in CT, specifically those with an impact on the imaging of cerebrovascular disease, are discussed in the remaining part of this chapter. The intent is to provide a summary of the clinical impact of each advance, offering guidance in terms of utility and day-to-day clinical implementation, with additional attention to radiation dose reduction.

This section is subdivided into six areas, all with clinical applicability. Although initially the innovations in these areas have been introduced only on high-end systems, with time this technology has been and will be translated to mid- and low-range cost systems. The topics covered include dual energy, iterative reconstruction, low kVp, perfusion imaging, radiation dose reduction, and new, innovative applications.

Technologic innovation continues in CT, involving the X-ray tube, detector, and image reconstruction, with major clinical impact. Achievements include increased spatial resolution, faster scan speeds, low kV (for reduced radiation/contrast agent dose), spectral prefiltration and advanced generation iterative reconstruction, morphologic and functional information from dual energy, and 4D CTA and perfusion with lower radiation dose.

Dual Energy

Established indications for dual energy CT are many and include virtual unenhanced images and direct bone subtraction. Imaging in dual energy mode can be routinely performed in the clinic, without additional radiation dose or compromise in image quality, in particular when the

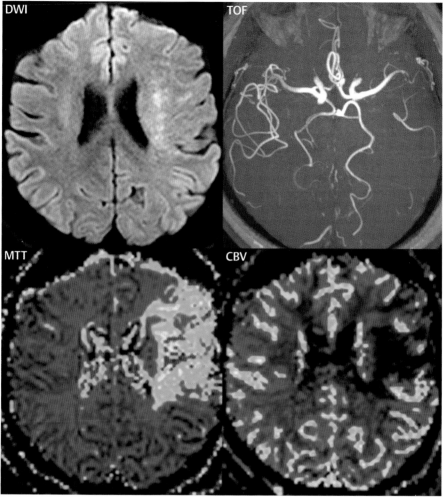

Fig. 1.19 Hyperacute middle cerebral artery infarct (with diffusion-perfusion mismatch and subsequent thrombectomy). Clinical presentation was within a few hours of symptom onset, with CT, MR, and DSA performed in a rapid temporal sequence. Unenhanced CT was normal, specifically without evidence of parenchymal hemorrhage (not shown). On the MR perfusion study, the area of ischemia (involving a portion of the left MCA distribution) is well identified on the MTT image, with a smaller region of reduced perfusion (CBV). Only a small area of abnormality involving the white matter of the corona radiata is noted on diffusion weighted imaging (with restricted diffusion, confirmed on the ADC map, not shown); thus there is a large diffusion-perfusion mismatch (representing the penumbra, or tissue at risk). There is also a paucity of left MCA branches on the TOF MRA, reflecting either occlusion or slow flow.

spectral separation is optimized by additional prefiltration of the high-energy X-ray beam. New-generation single-source CT scanners allow for sequential dual energy scans, a strategy that can be employed to extend dual energy metal artifact reduction to this class of scanners.

An additional important application with recent further developments is metal artifact reduction. Energetic extrapolation with dual energy dual source scanners has been shown to be an excellent strategy to reduce metal artifacts, regardless of the type of metal or implant (as long as the metallic objects are not too dense). Additional clinically significant findings can be evident with this approach.

Iterative Reconstruction (IR)

Iterative reconstruction techniques can be applied in CT, across the full range of exams, **21**

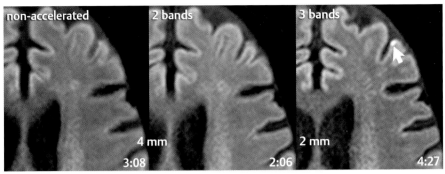

Fig. 1.20 Slice acceleration in combination with read-out segmentation, for improved infarct visualization on DWI at 3 T. In this example, rs-EPI scans without and with slice acceleration (using factors of 2 and 3) are compared. Image acquisition times are given in the lower right hand corner of each scan. In this example, by acquiring 2-mm sections (not possible without slice acceleration due to a very long scan time), a small cortical infarct is revealed (*white arrow*), which was not seen on 4-mm sections.

to reduce image noise. This improvement in image quality can be used to lower the radiation dose of CT exams. Current third-generation techniques combine statistical data modeling in the raw data domain with model-based noise reduction in the image domain. Using such techniques can lead to substantial dose reduction with little effect on image quality.

Low Peak Kilovoltage

Recent advances in X-ray tube design have allowed high power to be maintained at low kVp (for example, 1300 mA at 70 kVp), with a wide range of voltage settings provided (70–150 kVp). This enables low kVp scanning, which leads to improved iodinated contrast visualization in combination with a substantial

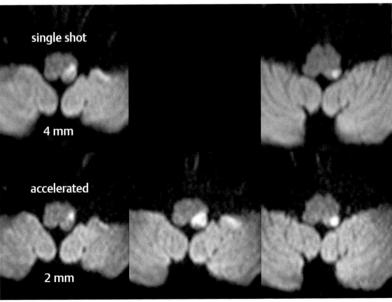

Fig. 1.21 Improved depiction of a lateral medullary infarct at 3 T by implementation of simultaneous multislice (slice accelerated) diffusion EPI. This infarct was visualized on two adjacent 4-mm sections using ss-EPI (upper row). Using simultaneous multislice technique, 2-mm sections can be acquired with only a minimal increase in scan time (1:32 vs 1:23 min:sec), resulting in less partial volume imaging (on each slice) and depiction of the infarct on three adjacent sections (lower row), as opposed to two. Note that on the 2-mm sections, the infarct is more sharply defined and there is an additional slice in between the two locations matching the 4-mm sections.

reduction in X-ray dose. In CT angiography of the brain, low kVp can be utilized with smaller amounts of iodinated contrast media, as well as with less radiation dose, still achieving improved arterial enhancement (SNR and CNR) and overall image quality.

Perfusion Imaging

With the increased power possible at low kVp (given the latest X-ray tube design), used in combination with improved detector designs (with reduced electronic noise), volume CT perfusion can be performed with a substantial reduction in radiation dose compared to prior generation CTs. An extended scan range is an additional important advance, with coverage of the entire brain now routine—a critical advance in the imaging of acute stroke. For disease entities where CT is the primary imaging modality (for example, acute infarction), acquisition of quantitative CT perfusion parameters provides relevant prognostic and treatment information. Parametric maps with rCBV, rCBF, and MTT are now routinely generated in clinical practice (**Fig. 1.22**). Widespread availability of CT perfusion today makes triage of patients presenting with clinical symptoms of ischemia possible, which is of critical importance relative to therapy. The availability of perfusion CT for this group of patients has also had other benefits, for example, improving detection of small ischemic lesions (**Fig. 1.23**).

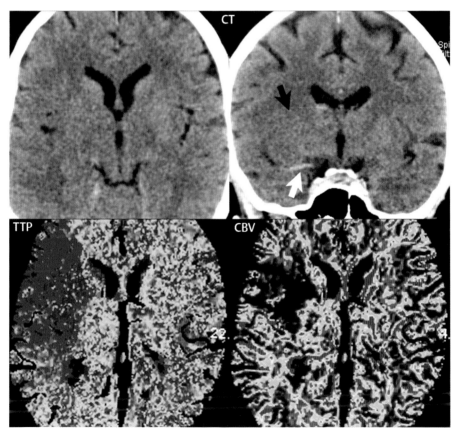

Fig. 1.22 Hyperacute middle cerebral artery infarct, with only subtle findings on conventional CT. There is mild hypodensity involving the right lentiform nucleus (seen both on the axial and coronal unenhanced CT, *black arrow*) together with a hyperdense right MCA sign (*white arrow*). A large hyperacute right MCA distribution infarct is readily evident on CBV and TTP maps, from the perfusion CT study, which has added a new dimension to the evaluation of ischemia since its clinical introduction more than a decade ago. There is a mismatch between the smaller core of infarcted tissue seen on the CBV study and the larger penumbra, or tissue at risk, as identified on the TTP map, suggesting that the lesion may be amenable in the acute setting to therapy.

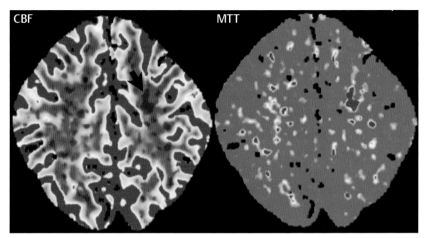

Fig. 1.23 Whole brain CT perfusion, now clinically available due to technologic innovations, improves diagnostic utility and also makes possible detection of small, acute brain infarcts. This is in addition to its use for the delineation of irreversibly infarcted tissue (versus the penumbra) in large cortical infarcts. The CT scans in this patient, specifically the CBF and MTT images, were acquired 1.5 hours following symptom onset and reveal a small ischemic lesion (*arrow*) in the left central semiovale (which was not seen on the conventional CT exam). The lesion was confirmed by MR (DWI), performed 2 days later (image not shown).

Reprinted with permission from Thierfelder KM, von Baumgarten L, Lochelt AC, et al. Diagnostic accuracy of whole-brain computed tomographic perfusion imaging in small-volume infarctions. Invest Radiol. 2014;49(4):236–242.

Radiation Dose Reduction

There are many important approaches to lowering radiation dose in CT, two of which have already been discussed—iterative reconstruction and low kVp. Of importance for brain is the use of lower kVp ($\leq$ 80) for CTA and perfusion, offering both lower radiation dose and higher sensitivity to iodinated contrast media. An additional important technique is the use of a tin filter. Tin filtering lowers dose by blocking low-energy photons, generated by the X-ray tube, from reaching the patient. In the latest generation CT, these and other methods are all used in concert, resulting in a markedly lower radiation dose while maintaining image quality. Of additional interest is radiation reduction in dose-sensitive organs, with a combination of techniques (including organ-based tube current modulation) routinely applied, for example, for lowering the dose to the thyroid and lens.

New and Innovative Applications

CT technology continues to evolve, focusing on radiation dose reduction with preserved image quality, together with increased speed and improved spatial resolution. The latest technology enables several new clinical applications and also improves the breadth of routine and specialty exams that are today the forte of CT. Pediatric imaging (which can be performed without sedation) and the imaging of uncooperative patients benefit greatly by the increased speed of current generation scanners.

New detector designs also offer improved spatial resolution. Current technology supports minimum slice widths of 0.4 mm and in-plane spatial resolution up to 32 line pairs/cm. Clinical applications include the temporal bone and other areas where bony detail is important. Not to be overlooked in these advances is the simplicity today, and clinical importance, of obtaining postprocessed images, whether these be simply sagittal and coronal reformatted images obtained from an axial acquisition or application of volume rendering techniques, for example in CTA.

Automated CT techniques, based on image processing alone or on the characterization of tissue using dual-energy CT, will eventually be a part of mainstream clinical practice, improving lesion detection and characterization. Automatic detection and volume estimation of infarcts, in particular acute infarcts that are quite subtle on CT, are currently well within the grasp of computer technology.

Another example is the limited ability of screening CT to differentiate between hemorrhage, iodinated contrast, and calcification, with dual energy offering a major advance in this role (**Fig. 1.24**). Color-coded CT

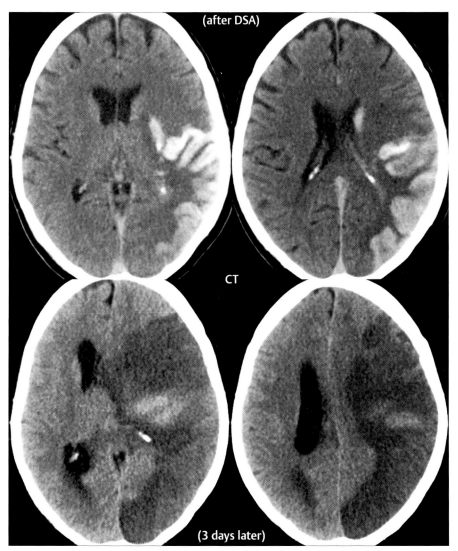

Fig. 1.24 Gyriform hyperdensity in a large left MCA and watershed territory infarct, due to prior DSA and not hemorrhage. The patient presented with signs of a large acute left MCA infarct and proceeded to DSA. The images on the top row were acquired within hours following DSA and show gyriform hyperdensity in the left MCA and watershed distributions, including the left caudate head. By imaging appearance alone, this could represent either hemorrhage or residual intravenous contrast (with blood-brain barrier disruption, as might be present in a massive early infarct). A follow-up CT obtained 3 days later proves the attenuation to be a result of iodine, due to its predominant clearance. There is also progression in low attenuation of the infarct itself and prominent mass effect with subfalcine herniation, increased intracranial pressure (reflected by the absence of sulci), and trapping of the right lateral ventricle. Today, dual energy CT plays a major role in this application, providing early and accurate discrimination between contrast extravasation and parenchymal hemorrhage, in particular in acute ischemic stroke patients who undergo DSA (and thrombolysis or clot removal).

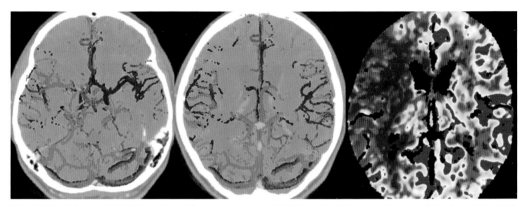

Fig. 1.25 Color-coded CT angiography, a recent innovation with applicability in acute infarction, is shown in a patient with an occlusion of the right internal carotid artery. At the two levels presented, there is delayed flow within the right MCA vessels, with collateralization via the anterior communicating artery to the MCA. From the CT perfusion study, CBF is markedly reduced as well in the right MCA territory.

Reprinted with permission from Thierfelder KM, Havla L, Beyer SE, et al. Color-coded cerebral computed tomographic angiography: Implementation of a convolution-based algorithm and first clinical evaluation in patients with acute ischemic stroke. Invest Radiol. 2015;50(5):361–365.

angiography, a new method of displaying dynamic cerebral CTA, provides the exam reader with important additional diagnostic information, including differentiation between ante- and retrograde flow and leptomeningeal collateralization (**Fig. 1.25**).

■ Summary

Advances in technology have speeded the evolution of both CT and MR as clinical modalities, a process made possible in part by the concurrent evolution of computers, enabling control of the scanners, data handling, and image reconstruction as we know it today. Much of the innovation has also been driven by the growing importance in clinical medicine of cross-sectional imaging for disease diagnosis and treatment evaluation.

Imaging of the brain today occupies a central role in medical care in regard to any question of CNS involvement or symptoms. This represents a marked change and a critical advance from 50 years ago, when diagnosis relied on plain radiographs, pneumoencephalography, and cerebral (X-ray–based) angiography.

2 Normal Anatomy

◼ Brain Parenchyma

The major divisions of the human brain include the cerebrum, cerebellum, and brainstem. The cerebrum is further subdivided into the frontal, parietal, occipital, and temporal lobes, and the insular cortex. The frontal lobe is separated posteriorly from the parietal lobe by the central sulcus. The sylvian fissure separates the frontal lobe from the temporal lobe inferiorly. There are lateral, polar (the most anterior region), orbital, and medial parts of the frontal lobe. Sulci of note include the central sulcus, which divides the precentral gyrus anteriorly (containing primary motor cortex) from the postcentral gyrus posteriorly (containing primary somatosensory cortex), the precentral sulcus (with the superior, middle, and inferior frontal gyri lying anteriorly, and the precentral gyrus posteriorly), the superior frontal sulcus (dividing the superior and middle frontal gyri), and the inferior frontal sulcus (dividing the middle and inferior frontal gyri). Broca's area, with functions related to speech production, lies in the dominant hemisphere (the left side, in right-handed individuals), within the pars opercularis and pars triangularis of the inferior frontal gyrus.

The parietal lobe lies behind the frontal lobe and is anterior and superior to the occipital lobe. The somatosensory cortex lies just posterior to the central sulcus within the postcentral gyrus, with the homunculus commonly used to illustrate the location therein of the different body regions (the homunculus is also used in reference to motor cortex). The sylvian fissure divides in part the parietal lobe from the temporal lobe inferiorly, with the parietal-occipital sulcus/fissure (seen medially) dividing those two respective lobes.

The occipital lobe contains the primary visual cortex, which lies medially within the calcarine sulcus. Above this sulcus is the cuneus, and below the lingual gyrus. The occipital lobe rests on the tentorium. There is no clear-cut division on the lateral surface of the brain between the occipital lobe and the neighboring parietal and temporal lobes. A theoretical dividing line can be drawn extending from the parieto-occipital fissure to the temporo-occipital incisure.

Within the medial temporal lobe lies the hippocampus, which is critical for memory formation. Within the temporal lobe are also areas for auditory and visual processing of sensory input. In the dominant hemisphere, the temporal lobe contains the primary auditory cortex, with Wernicke's area (critical for speech processing) located posteriorly in the superior temporal gyrus (Brodmann area 22).

The insular cortex (insula, or "island") is a portion of cerebral cortex folded deep within the sylvian fissure. Overlying the insula laterally is a cortical area termed the operculum, which includes parts of the frontal, temporal, and parietal lobes. The central sulcus of the insula divides the anterior part from the posterior part of the insula. Within the anterior insula, there are anterior, middle, and posterior short gyri (which converge to the apex anteriorly), and within the posterior insula, there are anterior and posterior long gyri.

The corpus callosum (CC) is the largest interhemispheric commissure in the brain. The CC is divided into the genu (the "knee") anteriorly, the body, and the splenium posteriorly. There is an additional small named segment, the rostrum (coming from the Latin and meaning "beak," as on a bird), which is a continuation of the genu and projects posteriorly and inferiorly.

Other links between the two cerebral hemispheres include the very small anterior and posterior commissures. The line connecting these two commissures, the AC-PC line, today defines the standard axial plane for MR acquisitions. These structures cannot be identified on CT, with the orbitomeatal line (OML)—connecting the lateral canthus of the orbit and the external auditory meatus—widely used to define the axial CT plane. This leads to difficulty in clinical comparison of axial MR and CT scans of the brain, with the two lines differing on average by slightly more than 10 degrees. Critical to image interpretation, and particularly valuable for imaging follow-up, are appropriate standardization and consistency in acquired and displayed imaging planes and axial tilt (**Fig. 2.1**).

The cerebellum lies in the posterior fossa, with the fourth ventricle, pons, and medulla anteriorly. Like the cerebrum, the cerebellum is divided into two hemispheres. However, in addition, there is a narrow midline zone, the vermis. The large folds of the cerebellum divide the structure into 10 smaller lobules. The primary fissure of the vermis divides that structure into anterior and posterior lobules. Readily recognizable anatomic portions of the

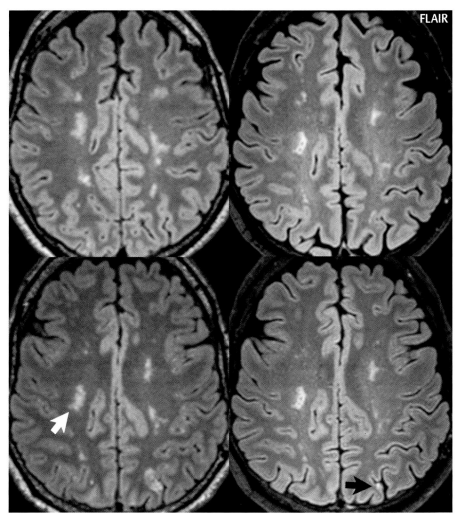

Fig. 2.1 Standardization of the axial imaging plane, enabling improved evaluation of follow-up exams. Watershed infarcts are presented on FLAIR images from an exam the week following clinical presentation (left column) and at 3 months (right column). The upper row of images are the original axial reformatted images from the 3D data sets, and the images in the lower row have been reformatted to match imaging plane for the two exams. Note that by standardization of the displayed imaging plane, the larger deep white matter infarct on the right (*white arrow*) can now be easily identified on the follow-up exam, and its evolution assessed, with gliosis replacing the previously identified edema, in a slightly smaller area of involvement, with central cavitation. Comparison of a cortical lesion in the superior parietal gyrus on the left (*black arrow*), now enabled by the standardization of the presented axial plane, reveals extensive resolution of edema with only a pinpoint area of gliosis remaining.

cerebellum on imaging include the nodulus (the anterior end of the inferior vermis, which projects into the fourth ventricle inferiorly like a thumb), the flocculus (a small lobule that is lateral to the medulla and inferior/medial to the internal auditory canals), and the cerebellar tonsil (a round lobule medially on the undersurface of the cerebellum). The cerebellar cortex itself is made up of very tightly folded layers, the folia. Although there are four deep cerebellar nuclei, the dentate nucleus is by far the largest and the only nucleus consistently recognized and described clinically on MR. The cerebellum plays a major role in motor control. The cerebellar peduncles connect the cerebellum to the brainstem. The superior and inferior cerebellar peduncles are small in size, with the middle cerebellar peduncle by far the largest.

The brainstem is composed of the midbrain, pons, and medulla oblongata. Cranial nerves III through XII originate from the brainstem, with nuclei of cranial nerves V through VIII within the pons. The two main components of the pons are the ventral (anterior) pons and the dorsal tegmentum. The ventral pons consists predominantly of white matter tracts with transverse fibers. The medulla has an anterior median fissure, with a raised area on either side, the pyramids (containing the pyramidal tracts). The swellings just lateral to the pyramids contain the inferior olivary nuclei. Axons of the corticospinal tract (motor) travel through the posterior limb of the internal capsule, thence through the cerebral peduncle anteriorly and into the anterior medulla (forming the pyramid medially). Below this prominence, the majority of axons cross to the opposite side. Other major tracts include the posterior (dorsal) column—medial lemniscus pathway (PCML, sensory—mechanoreceptors and proprioceptors) and the spinothalamic tract (sensory—nociceptors and thermoreceptors). Both convey information from the body to the postcentral gyrus. Neurons of the PCML travel within the dorsal column of the spinal cord, synapse in the medulla, cross over to the contralateral side of the medulla in the medial lemniscus, and ascend to the thalamus and subsequently to the somatosensory cortex. Neurons of the spinothalamic tract, after entering through the dorsal root (like the PCML),

synapse in the dorsal horn and then cross to the contralateral side of the spinal cord and ascend in the anterolateral quadrant through the brainstem to the thalamus, and from there to somatosensory cortex.

For more detail in terms of an anatomical atlas, the reader is referred to the many computer-based atlases, including *The Human Brain in 1969 Pieces* (Thieme, 2014).

■ Arterial Anatomy

Today, in the most widely used numbering system, there are seven recognized segments (C1 to C7) of the internal carotid artery (ICA): the cervical, petrous, lacerum, cavernous, clinoidal, ophthalmic, and communicating (terminal) segments. C1 (the cervical segment) extends from the carotid bifurcation to the skull base, with no branches. At its origin, the internal carotid artery is somewhat dilated, forming the carotid bulb. C2 (the petrous segment) has three sections, the ascending (vertical), genu (a 90-degree bend), and horizontal portions. Petrous ICA branches are uncommon. C3 (the lacerum segment) is short (1 cm), being that portion of the ICA passing over the foramen lacerum. C4 (the cavernous segment) is S-shaped and surrounded by the cavernous sinus, extending to the proximal dural ring. This segment is divided into the posterior vertical, posterior bend, horizontal, anterior bend, and anterior vertical portions. Prominent small branches of the cavernous ICA include the posterior trunk (the meningohypophyseal artery) and the lateral trunk. C5 (the clinoid segment) is a tiny wedge-shaped segment that extends between the proximal and distal dural rings, with this segment widest on its lateral aspect. The distal dural ring is incomplete medially, a region known as the carotid cave and a site for aneurysms. C6 (the ophthalmic segment) extends from the distal dural ring (thus being the most proximal intradural portion of the ICA) to the origin of the posterior communicating artery (PCOM). The ophthalmic artery arises anteriorly from C6, coursing laterally (**Fig. 2.2**).

Significant branches of the ophthalmic include the central retinal and lacrimal arteries. The superior hypophyseal artery also

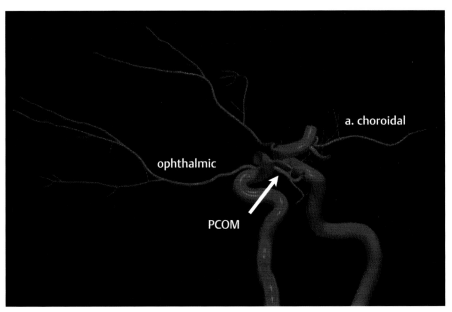

Fig. 2.2 Arterial branches from the C6 and C7 segments of the internal carotid artery. The ophthalmic artery arises from the anterior aspect of the C6 segment. The PCOM then arises posteriorly from the C7 segment. Just a few millimeters distally, the anterior choroidal artery arises from the posterolateral aspect of the C7 segment.

originates from C6, typically within 5 mm of the ophthalmic origin. C7 (the communicating segment) is that segment of the artery extending from just proximal to the origin of the posterior communicating artery to the carotid terminus, where the vessel divides into the anterior and middle cerebral arteries. C6 and C7 together constitute the supraclinoid internal carotid artery. The two major branches arising from the C7 segment are the PCOM and the anterior choroidal artery. A common variant is a persistent fetal origin, in which the PCOM is prominent, equal in diameter to the P2 segment of the posterior cerebral artery, with the P1 segment usually hypoplastic. Equally common is a hypoplastic PCOM. An infundibulum, a mild (< 3 mm) symmetric dilatation at the origin of the PCOM, is considered a normal variant. The anterior choroidal artery arises posteriorly laterally from the ICA, 2 to 4 mm distal to the PCOM, and supplies the posterior limb of the internal capsule and portions of the globus pallidus, thalamus, and midbrain.

Three major arteries supply the cerebral hemispheres. The anterior cerebral artery (ACA) supplies the anterior two-thirds of the medial cerebral surface and 1 cm of superior medial brain over the convexity (**Fig. 2.3**).

Three segments are defined, A1 from the ICA to the anterior communicating artery (ACOM), A2 from the ACOM to the origins of the pericallosal and callosomarginal arteries, and A3 the subsequent distal branches. An azygous anterior cerebral artery, with a single unpaired A2 segment arising from the A1 juncture, is present in less than 1%. An accessory or duplicated anterior cerebral artery leads to the appearance of three anterior cerebral arteries (specifically three A2 segments), two laterally and one midline. This may represent persistence of a primitive median artery and is much more common than an azygous ACA. The recurrent artery of Heubner, a large lenticulostriate artery, usually originates from A2 (but may originate from A1 or the ACA-ACOM junction) and supplies the caudate head, anterior limb of the internal capsule, and the anterior part of the putamen (**Fig. 2.4**). The posterior limb of the internal capsule and portions of the globus pallidus, thalamus, and cerebral peduncle are supplied, as previously stated, by the anterior choroidal artery, which arises from the communicating or terminal segment (C7) of the ICA. Occlusion of either of these vessels leads to a very distinctive, and not uncommon,

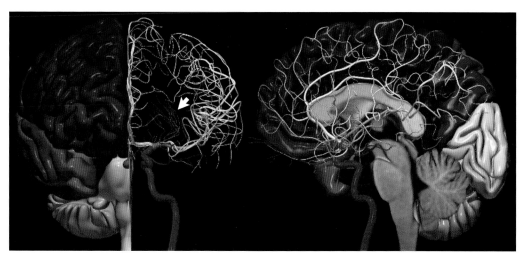

Fig. 2.3 The distal internal carotid artery and its major branches, the anterior and middle cerebral arteries. At the carotid terminus, the internal carotid artery divides into the anterior cerebral artery medially and the middle cerebral artery laterally. The distal branches of these two vessels supply the medial and anterolateral cortex. The lateral lenticulostriate arteries (*arrow*) arise from the M1 segment of the MCA and supply the basal ganglia and internal capsule.

presentation of infarction involving the basal ganglia and internal capsule.

The middle cerebral artery (MCA) supplies the lateral portion of the cerebral hemispheres, the insula, and the anterior and lateral temporal lobes (**Fig. 2.3**). Four segments are defined, with M1 from the carotid terminus to the bifurcation (trifurcation), M2 (with superior and inferior divisions) from the bifurcation to the circular sulcus of the insula, M3 (the opercular segments) from there to the superficial aspect of the sylvian fissure, and M4 the more distal cortical branches. Note that most anatomists (as opposed to clinicians) define M1 to extend slightly post-bifurcation. An MCA bifurcation is about three times more common than a trifurcation. Branches from M1 include the lateral lenticulostriate arteries and the anterior temporal artery (supplying the anterior temporal lobe). The former arise predominantly superiorly from the M1 segment, and supply the internal capsule, caudate nucleus, putamen, and globus pallidus. The origin of the anterior temporal artery is variable.

The posterior cerebral artery (PCA) supplies the occipital lobe and the medial temporal lobe. The PCA is commonly divided into four segments, with P1 from the basilar tip to the junction with the PCOM, P2 from the PCOM to the posterior aspect of the midbrain, P3 from there to the calcarine fissure, and P4 the subsequent terminal branches. The anterior thalamoperforators arise from the PCOM, and the posterior thalamoperforators arise from the P1 segment. The latter supply parts of the thalamus, brainstem, and posterior internal capsule. The thalamogeniculate arteries (also perforators) arise from the midportion of P2 and supply the posterior lateral thalamus, posterior limb of the internal capsule, and optic tracts.

The vertebral artery has four segments, V1 from its origin (along the posterior superior wall of the subclavian artery) to the foramen transversarium of C6, V2 from there to the foramen transversarium of C1, V3 from there to the dura, and V4 the distal intradural portion. Anomalous origins from the aortic arch occur.

Three major vessels supply the cerebellum. The posterior inferior cerebellar artery (PICA), the largest of these, originates from the V4 segment of the vertebral artery about 1.5 cm proximal to the vertebrobasilar junction. PICA supplies the lower medulla, cerebellar tonsils, inferior vermis, and posterior inferior cerebellar hemisphere (the inferior cerebellum with the exception of its most

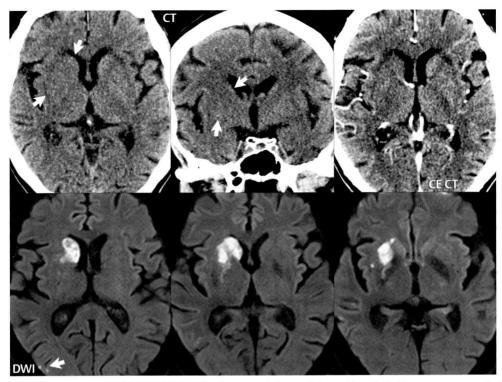

Fig. 2.4 Acute infarction of the caudate head and putamen. Two hours following initial clinical symptoms, there was no definite evidence of a focal low-density lesion on CT. On the perfusion study (not shown), MTT was prolonged in the right MCA territory. Close inspection of the axial and coronal precontrast scans shows subtle loss of definition of the right caudate head and the lentiform nucleus (*arrows*). On the CE CT, similar findings are evident. On MR, obtained 24 hours later, an acute infarct involving the caudate head, a portion of the anterior limb of the internal capsule, the putamen, and a small part of the globus pallidus is identified. Also present posteriorly (*white arrow*) are a few, very small, punctate cortical high SI foci, consistent with additional acute ischemic changes in a watershed territory. The recurrent artery of Heubner (also known as the medial striate artery) is the largest of the medial lenticulostriate arteries and arises in 90% of cases from the proximal A2 segment of the ACA. It supplies the caudate head, anterior lentiform nucleus, and anterior limb of the internal capsule, with involvement together of the caudate head and putamen (the striate nucleus) in ischemia as shown thus common.

anterior extent). PICA can be hypoplastic or absent (the latter in up to a quarter of cases). The vertebral artery may also terminate in PICA. The anterior spinal artery arises (bilaterally) from the vertebral artery distal to PICA and proximal to the vertebrobasilar junction.

The two vertebral arteries join to form the basilar artery near the level of the pontomedullary junction (**Fig. 2.5**). The basilar artery terminates near the pontomesencephalic junction. The anterior inferior cerebellar artery (AICA) arises from the basilar artery approximately 1 cm distal to the vertebrobasilar junction. AICA is the smallest of the three cerebellar arteries and supplies the anterior inferior portion of the cerebellum. It is commonly stated that the distribution of AICA is in equilibrium with PICA, with at times the distribution slightly larger or smaller. The superior cerebellar artery (SCA) arises from the basilar artery immediately prior to its termination. It supplies the superior half of the cerebellum. The SCA is not uncommonly duplicated. Extensive anastomoses exist between PICA, AICA, and the SCA. Basilar artery perforators arise throughout the length of the vessel and supply the brainstem. Medial perforators enter the pons near the midline, circumflex perforators travel a variable

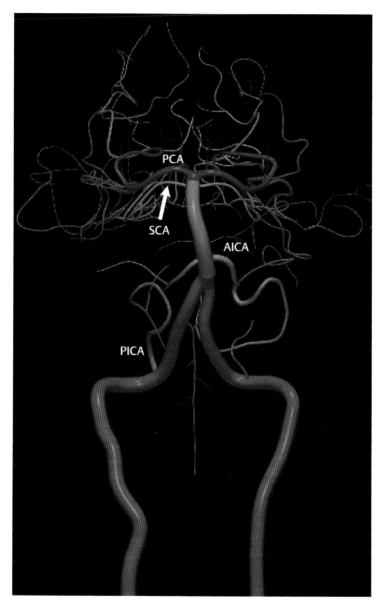

Fig. 2.5 The posterior circulation (the vertebrobasilar system). In this individual, on his right, as is most common, PICA arises from the distal vertebral artery, AICA from the proximal basilar artery, SCA from the distal basilar, and PCA from the termination of the basilar, with the relative sizes of the cerebellar vessels being PICA > SCA > AICA. However, the anatomy of the cerebellar vessels is highly variable, as illustrated on the patient's left, with PICA small and AICA compensating, being the dominant vessel of the three. Note that the anterior spinal artery is also visualized, originating bilaterally from the distal vertebral arteries (subsequent to the origin of PICA).

distance around the brainstem before entering. Fenestration of the basilar artery occurs in about 1%, with fenestrations of most of the proximal segments of the major arteries supplying the brain known (for example, the A1 and P1 segments), but less common.

The circle of Willis, the ring of connecting vessels providing important collateral circulation between the internal carotid arteries and the vertebrobasilar system, is well developed and symmetric in less than half of normal individuals. Asymmetry contributes to flow patterns that are important in the development of aneurysms and ischemic stroke. In half of normal individuals, at least one component is hypoplastic. The most common variant is a hypoplastic PCOM (about one-third of patients). A fetal origin PCA is seen in about 1 in 5 patients, typically with an accompanying hypoplastic P1 segment. A hypoplastic A1 is seen in about 1 in 10 patients. The ACOM, which connects the two anterior cerebral arteries, is hypoplastic in 5 to 15%.

The external carotid artery (ECA) is the smaller of the two terminal branches of the common carotid artery. It arises anterior and medial to the internal carotid artery, then courses posterior laterally. There are many muscular branches, with the early branching of the external carotid artery allowing rapid recognition of this vessel in distinction to the internal carotid artery. There are eight major branches, which can be grouped on the basis of their ventral or dorsal origin from the ECA. The ventral external carotid branches, in order by point of origin from proximal to distal, are the superior thyroid, lingual, facial, and internal maxillary arteries. The dorsal external carotid branches, similarly ordered, are the ascending pharyngeal, occipital, posterior auricular, and superficial temporal arteries. The middle meningeal artery arises from the internal maxillary artery.

There are numerous anastomoses between ECA branches and branches of the internal carotid and vertebral arteries, with three major anastomotic pathways described. In the orbital region, the internal maxillary and internal carotid circulations interface via the ophthalmic artery. Major interfaces also exist in the petrous-cavernous region and the upper cervical region, with the latter extending between the ascending pharyngeal or occipital artery and the vertebral artery. Pial-leptomeningeal anastomoses are very common and are an important potential source of collateral blood flow in occlusive vascular disease (**Fig. 2.6**).

There are also multiple internal carotid-vertebral/basilar artery anastomoses, which represent persistent embryonic circulatory patterns. One of these is seen not infrequently, as a normal variant, and is the persistent trigeminal artery. This vessel, when present, joins the proximal intracavernous segment of the internal carotid artery with the mid- or distal portion of the basilar artery. Presence of a persistent trigeminal artery is frequently associated with hypoplasia of the midsection of the basilar artery. A persistent hypoglossal artery is the second most common carotid-basilar anastomosis, arising from the internal carotid artery between the bifurcation and C1, and traversing the hypoglossal canal.

■ Venous Anatomy

Of the extracranial veins, the orbital veins are the most relevant to the subject of this text. The superior ophthalmic vein is the largest of these, with its normal flow posteriorly and medially to the cavernous sinus. It has anastomoses with the supraorbital vein and the angular vein. This is an important anastomosis between the intracranial and extracranial venous systems, with enlargement seen in the presence of a carotid-cavernous fistula.

The venous anatomy of the brain is highly variable. The intracranial venous sinuses are classically grouped into superior and inferior sets (**Fig. 2.7**). The superior group is composed of the vessels draining into the confluence of the sinuses (the torcular herophili) with subsequent drainage into the transverse and sigmoid sinuses. The superior sagittal sinus lies in the midline, originating near the crista galli and terminating at the torcula, with numerous bilateral (superficial convexity) cortical venous tributaries. The inferior sagittal sinus is much smaller and travels along the inferior border of the falx cerebri, draining into the straight sinus. The latter is formed by the confluence of the vein of Galen and the inferior sagittal sinus. The straight sinus drains posteriorly and inferiorly, underneath the splenium of the corpus callosum, and classically into the confluence of the sinuses. However, it can drain directly into a transverse sinus, typically the left. A small occipital sinus is present in slightly more than half of cases, traveling in the midline and draining superiorly into

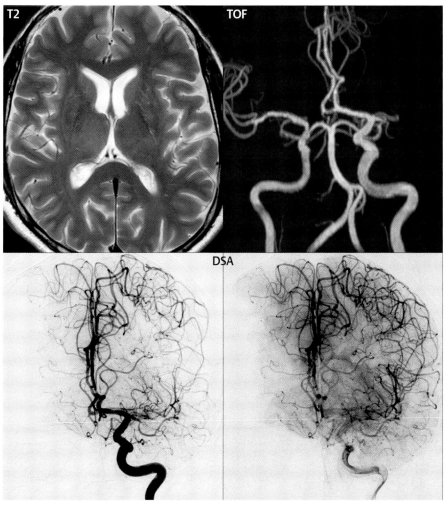

Fig. 2.6 Subtotal occlusion of the M1 segment of the left MCA, with excellent retrograde leptomeningeal collaterals. The patient was treated many years ago with balloon percutaneous transluminal angioplasty for an M1 stenosis on the left. On the T2-weighted scan, there is a subtle difference in caliber and number of visualized MCA branches when comparing the two sides. TOF MRA demonstrates apparent total occlusion of the left M1 segment just distal to the carotid terminus. Two different temporal phases from the frontal projection of the DSA are presented, with the second visualizing extensive collateral vascular supply to the left hemisphere. The patient was asymptomatic, despite the demonstrated occlusion.

the confluence of the sinuses. The latter, also termed the torcular herophili (or simply torcula), is formed by the junction of the superior sagittal, straight, transverse, and occipital sinuses. In a small number of cases, the superior sagittal sinus drains into one transverse sinus and there is no direct connection between the two transverse sinuses. The transverse sinuses travel within the peripheral margin of the tentorium, transitioning (in nomenclature) to the sigmoid sinuses when they leave the tentorial margin (at the base of the petrous temporal bone). The sigmoid sinus ends by definition at the jugular bulb, at the origin of the internal jugular vein. The transverse sinuses are commonly asymmetric, with the right typically larger. Arachnoid granulations are often visualized on MR within the transverse sinuses and can mimic a flow void due to a venous thrombus.

The inferior group of intracranial venous sinuses drains the lower brain surface,

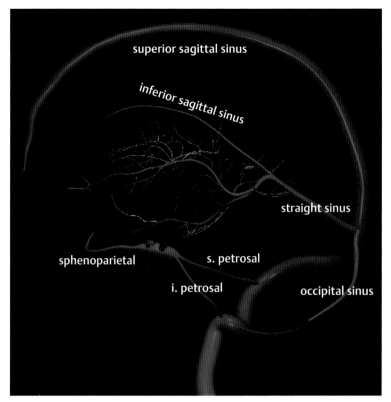

Fig. 2.7 The major venous sinuses of the brain. The superior sagittal sinus, straight sinus, and occipital sinus converge to the torcula, with subsequent drainage via the transverse and sigmoid sinuses to the internal jugular vein. Although not labeled, the major vessels of the deep venous system are evident, with the internal cerebral vein superiorly joining the basal vein of Rosenthal inferiorly to form the vein of Galen, which joins the inferior sagittal sinus to form the straight sinus. Anteriorly, the sphenoparietal sinus drains into the cavernous sinus. Posteriorly, the superior (s.) and inferior (i.) petrosal sinuses are seen, which both drain the cavernous sinus.

sylvian veins, and orbits. Its major components include the cavernous sinus, superior and inferior petrosal sinuses, sphenoparietal sinus, and basilar venous plexus. The superior petrosal sinus extends from the cavernous sinus to the transverse sinus, lying along the attachment of the tentorium to the petrous temporal bone. The inferior petrosal sinus connects the cavernous sinus and the jugular bulb, traveling in a groove between the clivus and the petrous apex. The sylvian veins drain via the sphenoparietal sinus into the cavernous, inferior petrosal, or transverse sinus. The basilar venous plexus extends over the dorsum of the clivus, connecting with the cavernous and inferior petrosal sinuses.

Supratentorial cortical veins include the sylvian (also known as the superficial middle cerebral vein), temporo-occipital, and superior convexity veins. These drain the cortex and subcortical white matter. The vein of Labbé is defined as the largest temporo-occipital vein, crossing the temporal lobe convexity and connecting the sylvian vein to the transverse sinus. The vein of Trolard is defined as the largest superior convexity vein connecting the sylvian vein and the superior sagittal sinus.

The periventricular white matter, basal ganglia, and thalamus are drained by the deep venous system (**Fig. 2.8**). The drainage is centripetally, as opposed to the drainage for the cortical venous system, which is centrifugally. Medullary veins drain the cerebral white matter, joining the subependymal veins. The thalamostriate vein joins the septal vein, posterior to the foramen of Monro, to form the

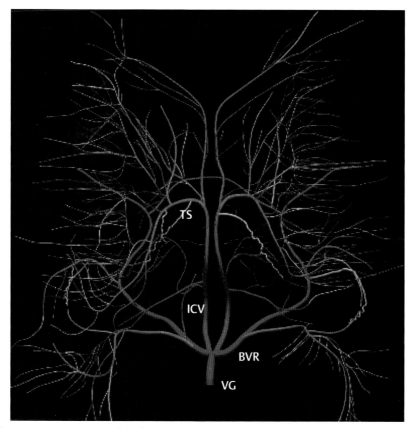

Fig. 2.8 The deep venous system of the brain. Seen in a craniocaudal projection, the thalamostriate veins (TS) drain bilaterally into the paired internal cerebral veins (ICV), which posteriorly join the basal veins of Rosenthal (BVR) to form the vein of Galen (VG).

internal cerebral vein. The paired basal veins of Rosenthal join the paired internal cerebral veins to form the vein of Galen. The vein of Rosenthal is the largest of the cisternal veins, and travels between the midbrain and the temporal lobe. The vein of Galen originates in the quadrigeminal cistern, running posterior-superiorly to the apex of the tentorium where it joins the straight sinus.

The venous system of the brain is best demonstrated by MR, as compared to CT. Techniques used for image acquisition include 2D TOF MRA, phase contrast MRA, and postcontrast scans including specifically 3D TOF MRA.

■ Common Anatomic Variants

The terms *Virchow-Robin space* and *perivascular space* are used interchangeably. This is a normal CSF space surrounding the perforating arteries entering the brain, and represents an invagination of the subarachnoid space. Dilated perivascular spaces are isodense on CT and isointense on MR, relative to CSF. There are three common locations in which dilated perivascular spaces are seen. The first location is within the inferior third of the lentiform nucleus. In this instance, the dilated spaces lie adjacent to the anterior commissure, following the course of the lateral lenticulostriate arteries. Although usually less than 5 mm in diameter, larger dilated perivascular spaces can be seen in this location. Differentiation can be difficult at times from chronic lacunar infarcts, with the latter the more common finding superiorly in the lentiform nucleus. The second common location for dilated perivascular spaces is within the white matter of the centrum semiovale. These follow the course of nutrient arteries, which lie along the white matter radiations. Thus, depending upon orientation relative to the slice, they may be seen either in cross-section or in plane, the latter as small radial structures. In the elderly, perivascular spaces may be more prominent (larger and more numerous), particularly in this location. The third site, which is less common than the other two, is in the cerebral peduncle (near the substantia nigra). Although bilateral lesions may be seen here, typically the lesion on one side is much larger than the other.

Arachnoid granulations are small focal areas of arachnoid that protrude through the dura into the venous sinuses of the brain. CSF exits from the subarachnoid space via arachnoid granulations and enters the bloodstream, in part due to the normal higher pressure of CSF. These granulations also function as one-way valves. As MR has improved in terms of image quality and spatial resolution, visualization of arachnoid granulations within the large dural sinuses, in particular the transverse sinuses, is not unusual. These should not be confused for venous thrombi.

3 Hemorrhage

■ Parenchymal Hemorrhage

Hemorrhage has a specific but varied appearance on MR, dependent on time frame. The appearance is much more straightforward on CT. In normotensive young adults, vascular malformations are the most common cause of spontaneous hemorrhage. In adults, parenchymal hemorrhage is most often due to hypertension (**Fig. 3.1**), whereas

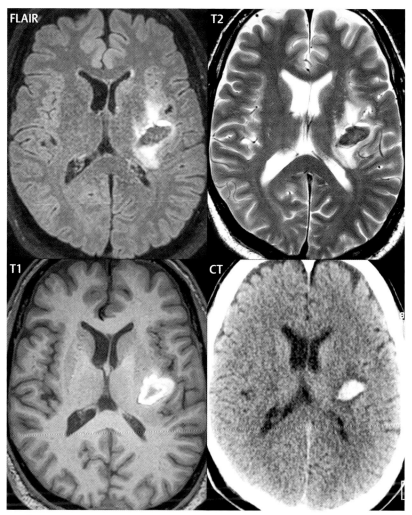

Fig. 3.1 Acute hypertensive hemorrhage. On MR, obtained 7 days following clinical presentation, a predominantly intracellular methemoglobin hemorrhage is seen on the left, with low signal intensity on the T2-weighted exam and high signal intensity on the T1-weighted scan. The hematoma extended superiorly from the globus pallidus and putamen. There is mild surrounding vasogenic edema. A small portion of the hemorrhage anteriorly is high signal intensity on the T2-weighted scans, consistent with an extracellular methemoglobin component. The CT obtained 1 day following presentation demonstrates the hematoma to be hyperdense, with mild surrounding low-density vasogenic edema.

subarachnoid hemorrhage is commonly due to rupture of an intracranial aneurysm. Typical locations for hypertensive hemorrhage include, in order of decreasing frequency, the basal ganglia (in particular, the putamen), thalamus, pons, and cerebellar hemisphere. The descriptions of the appearance of hemorrhage in the literature are predominantly for parenchymal bleeds. To some extent, the appearance of subarachnoid hemorrhage is similar.

Hyperacute hemorrhage on CT is of moderate density, rapidly increasing further in density (attenuation) over the first few hours due to clot formation and retraction. After a few days, in the subacute time frame, a progressive loss in attenuation begins. By 1 to 4 weeks, a hematoma will be isodense to brain, and in the chronic phase may appear hypodense.

The subsequent description of hemorrhage on MR is for the field strengths of 1.5 and 3 T, covering the vast majority of clinical systems today. Magnetic susceptibility effects (T2*), which cause decreased signal intensity depending on the time frame of the hemorrhage, are much less evident at lower field strengths.

On MR, hemorrhage follows a regular well-defined temporal progression of changes in signal intensity. Oxyhemoglobin (hyperacute) progresses to deoxyhemoglobin (acute), to intracellular methemoglobin (early subacute), then to extracellular methemoglobin (late subacute), and eventually to hemosiderin (chronic) (**Fig. 3.2**).

Oxyhemoglobin (hyperacute hemorrhage) has the signal intensity of fluid—high on T2- and low on T1-weighted scans. This imaging appearance is relatively nonspecific. Within hours, however, deoxyhemoglobin (acute hemorrhage) is evident with distinctive low signal intensity on T2-weighted scans. Deoxyhemoglobin does not have a unique appearance on T1-weighted scans, on which it appears isointense to mildly hypointense. Methemoglobin (subacute hemorrhage) has distinctive high signal intensity on T1-weighted scans, and bleeds can be further subdivided temporally into intracellular and extracellular methemoglobin. Initially, in the intracellular phase, blood will be high signal intensity on a T1-weighted scan and low signal intensity on a T2-weighted scan (the latter due to a susceptibility effect). With red blood cell lysis, methemoglobin becomes

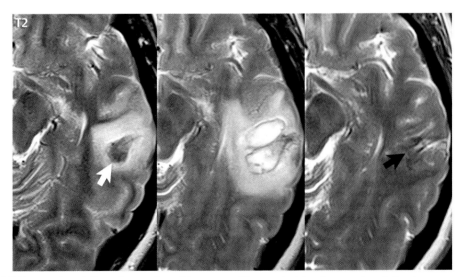

Fig. 3.2 Temporal evolution of parenchymal hemorrhage on MR. On initial presentation, this posterior temporal hematoma (*white arrow*) demonstrates low signal intensity on the T2-weighted scan, indicative of deoxyhemoglobin. Also present is surrounding vasogenic edema, with abnormal high signal intensity. Two weeks later, temporal evolution has occurred to extracellular methemoglobin, with high signal intensity on the T2-weighted scan. Five months following presentation, there has been resorption of most of the fluid, together with resolution of the edema, leaving a low signal intensity hemosiderin cleft (*black arrow*).

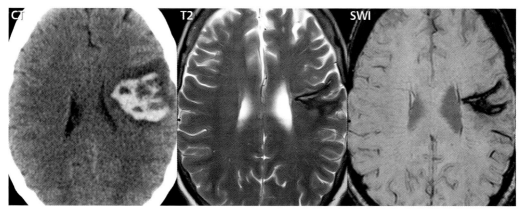

Fig. 3.3 Parenchymal hemorrhage; temporal evolution from acute on CT to chronic on MR. In this lung transplant patient, a large acute parenchymal hematoma with mild surrounding vasogenic edema is noted in the left corona radiata on the initial CT. On the follow-up MR 2 years later, there is near complete resorption of the fluid centrally, with residual hemosiderin (abnormal low signal intensity) at the periphery. There is improved depiction of the hemosiderin on SWI.

extracellular in location, with distinctive high signal intensity on both T1- and T2-weighted scans. With time, methemoglobin is converted into hemosiderin, with chronic hemorrhage thus exhibiting pronounced low signal intensity on T2-weighted scans again due to susceptibility effects. The appearance of a chronic parenchymal hemorrhage on MR also depends on whether the central fluid collection is resorbed or not. If resorbed, a hemosiderin cleft will be left (**Fig. 3.3**).

If not resorbed, there will be a central fluid collection with high signal intensity on both T1- and T2-weighted scans, surrounded by a hemosiderin rim. With the passage of years, the fluid collection may change in appearance on T1-weighted scans from high to low signal intensity. Although the appearance of chronic hemorrhage on MR, with low signal intensity on T2-weighted scans, is generally well known, the relative sensitivity of different pulse sequences is often not as well understood (**Fig. 3.4**). It is important to note that the evolution of parenchymal hemorrhage on MR does not always follow the characteristic pattern described. Additional factors can be very important, including dilution, clotting, and hematocrit. One key to the recognition of parenchymal hemorrhage, not discussed in detail, is the presence of edema surrounding the hematoma, which is seen

in the hyperacute, acute, and early subacute stages.

■ Subarachnoid Hemorrhage

The appearance of acute subarachnoid hemorrhage on CT is generally well known, being well visualized with abnormal high attenuation (**Fig. 3.5**). Depending on the amount of blood present, the sensitivity for detection of subarachnoid hemorrhage on CT can decrease rapidly with time following presentation. CT can be negative in patients with subarachnoid hemorrhage due either to a time delay (a few days) between the hemorrhage and imaging or the small quantity of blood present.

MR is more sensitive for subarachnoid hemorrhage than CT, although the imaging appearance is complex and recognition thus more difficult, particularly for physicians with less experience (**Fig. 3.6**). FLAIR is extremely sensitive to changes in the CSF; thus even very small amounts of subarachnoid hemorrhage will be seen as abnormal high signal intensity within the sulci. However, this appearance is not specific for subarachnoid hemorrhage and can be seen in any disease process that leads to a subtle change from normal in the composition of CSF. Meningitis produces this appearance (high signal intensity within the

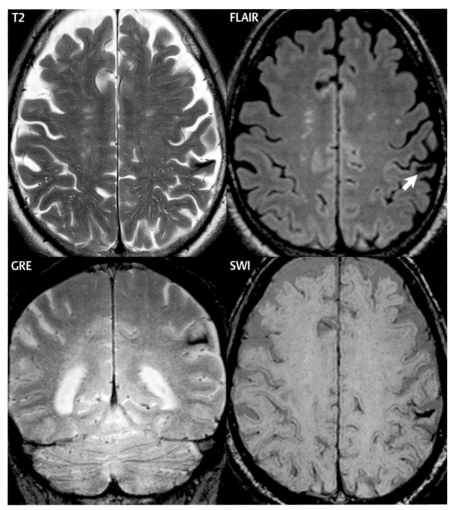

Fig. 3.4 Hemosiderin, within the supramarginal gyrus. The appearance of hemosiderin, the end product of chronic hemorrhage, is depicted on four MR scan techniques with differing sensitivity. Both T2-weighted FSE and FLAIR scans are relatively sensitive to the presence of hemosiderin on scans at 3 T, with a linear region of low signal intensity seen (*arrow*) within the supramarginal gyrus on the left on both scans. The better depiction on FLAIR in this instance is likely due to the thinner slice thickness (1 vs 4 mm), with less partial volume imaging. 2D GRE T2*-weighted scans are often used as a fast acquisition to detect hemorrhage (specifically either deoxyhemoglobin or hemosiderin) and are more sensitive than FSE T2-weighted scans or FLAIR. The GRE scan presented was obtained in the coronal plane, a common choice that offers additional visualization of the brain in a supplemental plane. The technique most sensitive to hemosiderin is susceptibility weighted imaging (SWI), which is typically acquired as a thin section 3D acquisition and requires a relatively long scan time.

sulci on FLAIR), and administration of 100% O_2 in ventilated patients is another known cause. Regional versus global distribution of changes on FLAIR aids in differentiation of these processes.

On T2* (susceptibility)-weighted images on MR, acute subarachnoid blood will be seen as low signal intensity, in distinction to normal high signal intensity CSF. In combination with the appearance on FLAIR, this finding is specific for acute subarachnoid hemorrhage. Depending on the time frame and the amount of hemorrhage, subarachnoid hemorrhage can also be seen as high signal intensity on

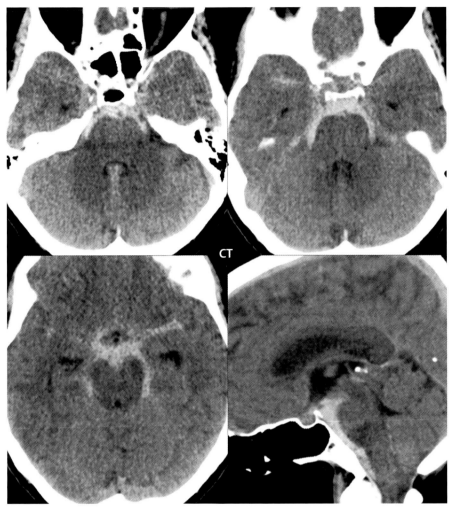

Fig. 3.5 Nontraumatic, spontaneous (nonaneurysmal) subarachnoid hemorrhage. The patient presented acutely with a severe headache, nausea, and vomiting. Three axial images and a sagittal reformatted image are presented. There is prominent, acute subarachnoid hemorrhage, confined to the midbrain cisterns (perimesencephalic). Only a tiny amount of intraventricular hemorrhage was noted (in the right atrium, not shown), and there was no parenchymal hemorrhage. No aneurysm was found on DSA, with a follow-up MR also negative. A ventricular shunt was not required, and patient recovery was uneventful.

T1-weighted scans, due to the presence of methemoglobin. By 3 days following presentation, high signal intensity is commonly seen on T1-weighted scans, a finding that typically persists for days to weeks. Subsequent to that time frame, and persisting long term, the residua of subarachnoid hemorrhage will be well seen on T2*-weighted images. In comparison, the sensitivity of CT to subarachnoid hemorrhage decreases markedly following the first few days, with CT often normal thereafter (**Fig. 3.7**).

Hemorrhage within the ventricular system is similarly well seen: in the acute time frame by CT, and regardless of time frame by MR. Blood clots are common within the ventricular system, with hyperdensity on CT and a variable but characteristic appearance on MR depending on composition. Layering of a small amount of hemorrhage posteriorly in the atria of the lateral ventricles is commonly visualized on MR, a finding that can persist for days to weeks following hemorrhage.

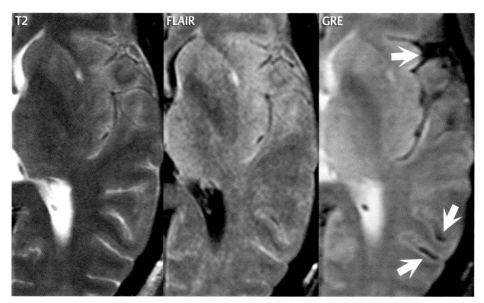

Fig. 3.6 Acute subarachnoid hemorrhage, MR. On initial inspection, the T2-weighted scan appears normal (other than a small external capsule chronic lacunar infarct). However, in retrospect (particularly in comparison with the GRE scan), the left sylvian fissure does not demonstrate the characteristic high SI of CSF (it is isointense with brain), raising the suspicion of subarachnoid hemorrhage or other pathology. FLAIR confirms this finding, but also demonstrates abnormal high SI in two sulci posteriorly, indicative of either blood or inflammatory changes. The GRE scan confirms that both findings represent subarachnoid hemorrhage (*arrows*), with abnormal low signal intensity due to T2* changes (seen with both deoxyhemoglobin and intracellular methemoglobin).

■ Superficial Siderosis

In superficial siderosis, there is hemosiderin deposition in macrophages within the membranes lining the CSF spaces. The cause is recurrent subarachnoid hemorrhage, typically due to a hemorrhagic neoplasm, ruptured aneurysm, or vascular malformation that has bled. The surface of the cerebellum is the most common site. Clinical symptoms occur infrequently, and only when there is substantial deposition of hemosiderin. Possible symptoms include sensorineural hearing loss, pyramidal tract signs, and cerebellar dysfunction, together with cranial nerve dysfunction (most often cranial nerves II, V, VII, or VIII, with the severity of injury proportional to the cisternal length of the nerve).

T2-weighted scans demonstrate hypointensity of the involved leptomeninges or ependyma. Any sequence that improves the sensitivity to susceptibility (T2*), such as a gradient echo sequence or susceptibility weighted imaging, will also be more sensitive to the presence of superficial siderosis (as well as the use of 3 T as opposed to 1.5 T). Subependymal siderosis is included within the more general category of superficial siderosis and can be seen secondary to neonatal intraventricular hemorrhage. The latter finding was described early in the development of higher field (≥ 1.5 T) MR systems, due to the greater sensitivity to T2* effects and specifically hemosiderin at higher field strengths (**Fig. 3.8**).

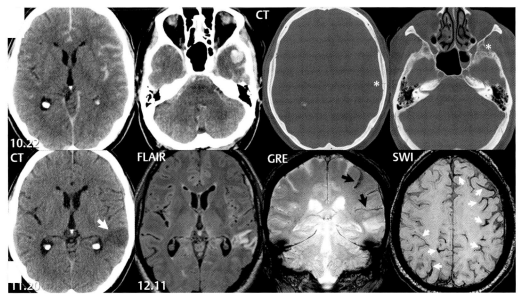

Fig. 3.7 Posttraumatic subarachnoid hemorrhage and infarction. On the initial CT, there is prominent subarachnoid hemorrhage most notably within the sylvian fissure on the left and along the falx anteriorly. At the level of the pons, subarachnoid blood is noted within the prepontine cistern, with an acute parenchymal hemorrhage also seen within the anterior inferior temporal lobe on the left. On the axial CT sections reconstructed with a bone algorithm, both temporoparietal (involving the convexity) and temporal sphenoid (along the anterior/inferior portion of the middle cranial fossa) fractures (*asterisks*) are noted. The former was comminuted and lies adjacent to the subsequently identified infarct, which was presumably posttraumatic, in the left temporoparietal region (*arrow*, CT of 11.20). The latter fracture lay adjacent to the parenchymal hemorrhage within the anterior temporal lobe. Subarachnoid hemorrhage is no longer visible on the follow-up CT 1 month after trauma. Note also the air-fluid level in the left major air cell of the sphenoid sinus at presentation, reflecting hemorrhage within the sinus. On the MR, obtained 2 months following trauma, gliosis in the area of the infarct is identified both on the axial FLAIR and the coronal T2*-weighted GRE images. There is extensive hemosiderin lining multiple gyri, the residua of subarachnoid hemorrhage, seen in part on the GRE image (*black arrows*) but much more evident on SWI (*small white arrows*). On the latter image, the hemosiderin is easily identified by comparison of the signal intensity within a normal sulcus (for example, within the anterior right frontal lobe), with that along the surface of the brain within an involved sulcus.

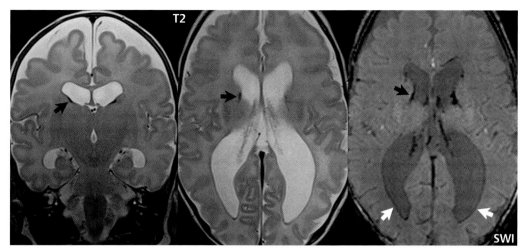

Fig. 3.8 Obstructive hydrocephalus, extraventricular (communicating hydrocephalus) in a 3-month-old infant following ventricular hemorrhage, evaluated on imaging at 3 T. The lateral ventricles are enlarged. The incidence of intraventricular hemorrhage is 20% in very-low-birth-weight premature infants (< 1500 g), with the patient illustrated born at 27 weeks with a weight of 940 g. Intraventricular hemorrhage begins in the periventricular germinal matrix, which lies in the caudothalamic groove. When the hemorrhage is substantial, blood enters the ventricular system. In this infant, the residua of hemorrhage (hemosiderin, *black arrows*) are seen on coronal and axial T2-weighted scans bilaterally at the caudothalamic groove. There is improved depiction of hemosiderin, with low signal intensity, in this location (*black arrow*) as well as along the ependyma of the occipital horns of the lateral ventricles (*white arrows*) on SWI.

4 Ischemia

■ Introduction

In younger patients, the etiologies for cerebral infarction are many and varied, in distinction to older adults (**Fig. 4.1**). Leading causes include cardiac and hematologic disease, infection, vasculitis, trauma, and illicit drug use. In the elderly, infarcts are most often due to atherosclerosis, with vessel occlusion due to either thrombosis or embolism. Common areas of atherosclerotic involvement include the carotid bifurcation, distal internal carotid artery, and middle cerebral artery. Risk factors for infarction in an adult include high blood pressure, high cholesterol, smoking, diabetes, obesity, cardiovascular disease, oral

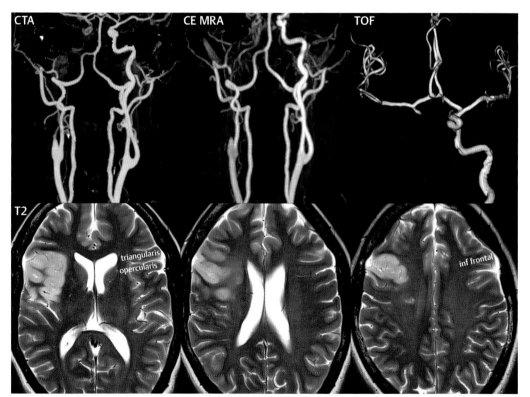

Fig. 4.1 MCA infarct due to cervical spinal manipulation in a younger adult. The T2-weighted axial exam depicts vasogenic edema (a subacute infarct, on the right) involving the anterior insula and inferior frontal gyrus, specifically including the pars triangularis and pars opercularis therein. CTA performed on admission 5 days prior to the MR reveals occlusion of the right internal carotid artery in its midsection, with a sharply tapered origin consistent with a dissection. By the time of the CE-MRA, the occlusion progressed to the level of the origin of the ICA. There is retrograde filling of the distal segment of the ICA seen both on the initial CTA and on the TOF MRA. On the CTA, this is demonstrated to extend to the level of the cavernous carotid artery, supplying the ophthalmic artery. Cerebral infarcts are known to occur in younger patients following high-velocity, low-amplitude cervical manipulation, due to both vertebral and internal carotid artery dissections.

contraceptives, and cocaine. Clinical presentations include acute neurologic deficit, speech disorder (aphasia), change in mental status, headache, and seizure.

Infarction involving the precentral gyrus (primary motor cortex) leads to contralateral motor deficits. Infarction in the left inferior frontal gyrus (specifically in Broca's area, the part of the brain responsible for speech production) causes an expressive aphasia. Infarction in the left posterior superior temporal gyrus (specifically in Wernicke's area) causes receptive aphasia. The latter two statements apply for patients who are left hemisphere dominant.

■ Acute Cerebral Ischemia

Imaging, whether by CT or MR, is today an essential part of stroke detection and decision making. There is great variability from institution to institution in regard to imaging protocols, in part dependent upon the available imaging technology. However, the time since symptom onset is very important in terms of the imaging approach. In the emergent setting at tertiary care centers, both CT and MR are readily available, with performance of at least one of these scans being a requisite prior to neuro-intervention.

In acute stroke triage, there are several questions that need to be answered rapidly and accurately by imaging. Does the scan identify a stroke, or is the clinical diagnosis possibly not correct? Is intracranial hemorrhage present? Is there occlusion of a major cerebral vessel? Is there a clinically relevant ischemic penumbra that is potentially salvageable? The latter also requires identification of irreversibly injured brain.

Stroke is a generic term signifying a neurologic event. Cerebral ischemia and cerebral infarction refer to the tissue status and can be assessed by CT and MR. Brain tissue remains potentially viable in cerebral ischemia, although blood flow is inadequate. In cerebral infarction, there is actual cell death. Time is critical in patient triage. The terms *hyperacute* and *acute* stroke are commonly used, although their definition varies from site to

site. In general, hyperacute refers to presentation within 6 hours following symptom onset. Use of the term *acute* is much more variable, although it is commonly employed for the patient who is within 6 to 48 hours from symptom onset.

There are three major etiologies for stroke:

1. The most common cause of acute ischemia is atherosclerosis, representing slightly less than half of all cases. Most large arterial infarcts are embolic, from thrombi originating at the site of an atherosclerotic plaque. The most common site for an embolus to lodge is just subsequent to the internal carotid artery terminus, in the middle cerebral artery, with occlusion of the vessel or a branch therein.

2. Small vessel disease accounts for a quarter of all strokes. Occlusion of small arteries generally results in lacunar infarcts, which are small, less than 2 cm in diameter. Many lacunar infarcts are clinically silent. Those located in strategic areas cause significant neurologic impairment. Most lacunar infarcts involve penetrating arteries, commonly in the basal ganglia (caudate nucleus, putamen, and globus pallidus), thalami, internal capsule, pons, and deep cerebral white matter.

3. Cardioembolic disease causes slightly less than one-quarter of all major strokes. Risk factors include myocardial infarction, arrhythmia (often atrial fibrillation), and valvular disease.

By location, the MCA is the most common site of large artery thromboembolic infarction, followed by the PCA, and then the vertebrobasilar circulation. The ACA territory is least commonly involved. Acute infarcts can be solitary or multiple. They vary in size from very small lacunar infarcts to large territorial lesions. When a large vessel is occluded by clot, involvement of peripheral secondary branches is common, with or without distal emboli. Ischemia is multifactorial, with hypertension, diabetes, smoking, obesity, and high serum triglycerides the known major risk factors.

In the center of an area of ischemia (the core), cerebral blood flow (CBF) falls precipitously. Oxygen is rapidly depleted and the cells die, with irreversible loss of function. In about half of patients, an ischemic penumbra surrounds this core. Here, CBF is substantially reduced, falling from a normal of 60 cm^3/100 g/min to 10 to 20 cm^3/100 g/min. Tissue in this region is at risk, but potentially salvageable. There is a hierarchy among cell types in the brain in terms of sensitivity to ischemic damage, with neurons most vulnerable. Neurons in certain areas of the brain are also more vulnerable to ischemia than those in other regions.

In the first 6 hours or so, gross changes (pathologically) involving the brain are minimal. This is reflected on MR by the lack of vasogenic edema (which is best seen by T2-weighted scans, and specifically FLAIR), without a bulk change in water. Cell swelling does, however, occur almost immediately, specifically cytotoxic edema, resulting in diffusion weighted imaging (DWI) being positive within minutes after the onset of ischemia. Gray-white matter boundaries become less distinct early on gross pathology, a finding that is also reflected by MR on T1- and T2-weighted sequences. With time, the gyri expand, compressing the adjacent sulci and effacing the adjacent CSF spaces.

Most infarcts occur in older adults. Children who present with an infarct typically have an underlying disease, for example sickle cell disease or a right-to-left cardiac shunt. Common causes in young adults include dissection and drug abuse. Clinical presentation includes sudden onset of a focal neurologic deficit and decreased consciousness. Prognosis depends on which vessel is occluded, collateral blood flow, and whether there is a significant ischemic penumbra.

Time is of the essence for successful treatment of acute stroke. Treatment options continue to evolve, together with inclusion and exclusion criteria. Critical considerations for successful intervention include time from symptom onset and the imaging findings on the screening exam. CT is most often employed, as opposed to MR, due to the need for the exam to be completed rapidly. Treatment using intravenous (IV) recombinant tissue plasminogen activator (rtPA) is usually reserved for lesions less than 3 hours in age, and intra-arterial thrombolysis is used for those less than 6 hours.

IV thrombolysis with rtPA (alteplase) unequivocally results in more patients with a favorable neurologic outcome (**Fig. 4.2**), although there is an increase in early fatal cerebral hemorrhages. Clinical trials have shown that hemorrhagic risk is clearly increased by administration of a thrombolytic agent, specifically alteplase. The spectrum seen ranges from frequent benign petechial hemorrhages to rare large hematomas (**Fig. 4.3**).

However, only the large parenchymal hematomas with mass effect are independently associated with clinical deterioration (**Fig. 4.4**). Time is critical regardless, with results best when given within 3 hours for IV thrombolysis (**Fig. 4.5**). Generally accepted imaging criteria for intra-arterial thrombolysis include a significant perfusion-diffusion mismatch (ischemic penumbra), involvement of less than one-third of the MCA territory, and the absence of parenchymal hemorrhage.

Endovascular mechanical thrombectomy is now also widely used, either as an alternative or with thrombolysis (**Fig. 4.6**). Certain patients, however, are not good candidates for thrombectomy (or other neuro-intervention, such as stent placement) (**Fig. 4.7**), in particular patients with very large infarcts. Infarct and penumbra size are critical for patient selection and correlate with functional outcome.

The following imaging approach is typically performed emergently in a patient presenting clinically with a stroke. A nonenhanced CT (NECT) is first performed. This is used to exclude parenchymal hemorrhage as well as other disease processes that may clinically mimic a stroke. A second critical issue is to determine whether a major cerebral vessel is occluded, with CT angiography (CTA) thus performed (typically from the aortic arch to the vertex). The third and final critical issue is to determine what part of the brain is

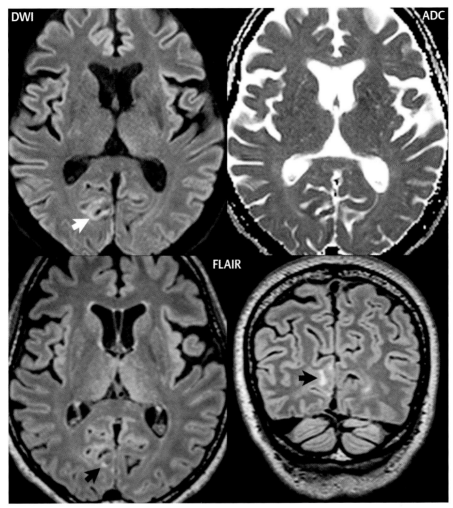

Fig. 4.2 Resolution of stroke symptoms following IV thrombolysis. In the cortex adjacent to the calcarine sulcus (*white arrow*) and in the cuneus (*black arrows*) are small areas with both restricted diffusion (high SI on DWI, with corresponding low ADC) and vasogenic edema. The MR was obtained 4 hours after symptom onset, with IV thrombolysis (rtPA) begun 1 hour later. At onset, a left homonymous hemianopsia was present that resolved by the time of hospital discharge.

irreversibly damaged and whether there is a clinically relevant ischemic penumbra. This is typically accomplished using perfusion CT (which requires a separate smaller dose of iodinated contrast, given at a high flow rate), although MR can also be employed. It should be noted that current generation CT scanners easily obtain perfusion maps of the entire brain, with the exam not limited to a small anatomic region (slab) as in the past.

Although acute ischemic strokes are often not detectable on initial NECT, careful image inspection is mandated. A dense MCA sign (due to acute thrombosis) is seen in about one-third of cases of M1 occlusion. The gray-white matter interface may be indistinct in the area of infarction. Relatively common findings, assuming that the relevant portion of the brain is involved, include loss of visualization of the insular cortex/ribbon and decreased density (with loss of definition) of the basal ganglia. In very large infarcts, there may be wedge-shaped, subtle parenchymal hypodensity together with subtle cortical sulcal effacement.

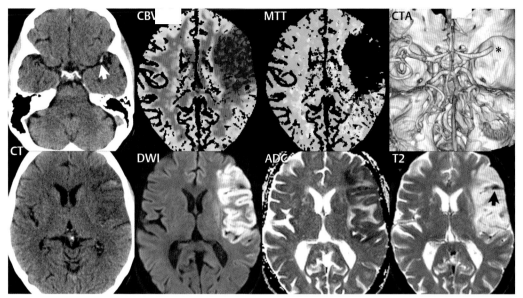

Fig. 4.3 Acute MCA occlusion, with no mismatch between the infarct core and ischemic penumbra. On the CT performed 5 hours after onset of symptoms, hyperdense thrombus (*white arrow*) is identified in the distal left M1 segment of the MCA. Although the infarct could not be identified on the basis of decreased attenuation, due to the early time frame, it is easily visualized on the basis of the CBV and MTT images. These reveal a large left MCA territory infarct, with no mismatch (the involved territory on both scans is very similar). CTA demonstrates occlusion of the M1 segment of the left MCA (*asterisk*). IV thrombolysis was begun at that time. One day later, the follow-up CT (lower row) reveals low density in the region, consistent with the development of vasogenic edema, but also a small hyperdense area within the infarct reflecting parenchymal hemorrhage. DWI confirms the large MCA distribution infarct, which involved the medial and inferior frontal gyri, the pre- and postcentral gyri, and the insula. Restricted diffusion is demonstrated on the ADC map. The patient was uncooperative, and thus the T2*-weighted b = 0 image from the echo planar DWI scan was used to identify early parenchymal hemorrhage, with the presence of deoxyhemoglobin (*black arrow*) confirmed in a similar distribution as that seen on CT. In acute stroke patients treated with IV tissue plasminogen activator, hemorrhagic transformation is seen in 40% and parenchymal hemorrhage in 10%.

CTA quickly answers the question of whether a major vessel occlusion is present. Perfusion CT (pCT) depicts the effect of the vessel occlusion on the brain parenchyma. Three parameter maps are classically calculated from pCT: cerebral blood volume (CBV), cerebral blood flow (CBF), and mean transit time (MTT). CBV is defined as the volume of blood present at a given moment within the brain (or a region therein). CBF is defined as the volume of blood flow to the brain in a given period of time. MTT is defined as the time necessary for blood to transit through a given brain volume. They are related mathematically by the following equation: CBF = CBV/MTT. On both CT and MR, these parameters are commonly depicted visually using a color scale, with numerical values also readily accessible. In normal brain, CBV and CBF are higher in gray matter as compared to white matter. Ischemic brain displays a slower transit time. The ischemic penumbra is the area of brain with moderately decreased CBF, but near-normal CBV, that surrounds the infarct core, the latter demonstrating markedly reduced CBF and CBV. Both the core and the ischemic penumbra demonstrate prolonged MTT. A caveat, however, is that extra- or intracranial stenosis can also cause decreased or delayed perfusion.

As described earlier, CT perfusion is performed to determine the mismatch

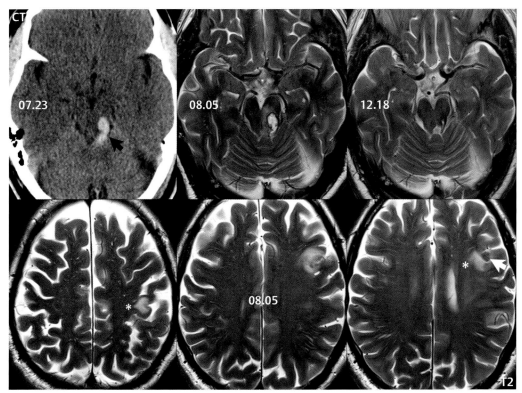

Fig. 4.4 Parenchymal hemorrhage, distant from the area of infarction, as a complication of IV thrombolytic therapy. The patient presented with symptoms of an acute left MCA distribution infarct, including aphasia and right upper extremity weakness. No hemorrhage was noted on the initial CT (not shown), with IV thrombolysis begun 3 hours following symptom onset. The CT presented, from 07.23, was performed 3.5 hours following administration of rtPA and reveals an acute parenchymal hemorrhage (*black arrow*) involving the left cerebral peduncle and inferior colliculus. The MR performed 2 weeks later better depicts the involvement of the brainstem, with the hemorrhage high SI, consistent with extracellular methemoglobin. The hemorrhage was also high SI at this time point on the T1-weighted scan (not shown). A thin rim of hemosiderin is already present on the T2-weighted scan, and there is extensive edema surrounding the hemorrhage within the left cerebral peduncle. A further follow-up MR, 4 months later, revealed as the residua of this hemorrhage a small fluid cleft, mild hemosiderin deposition, and focal atrophy. The lower row of images depicts a portion of the initial infarct, with vasogenic edema noted within the pre- and postcentral gyri (*asterisks*). Note also the occurrence of a second parenchymal hemorrhage (*white arrow*, deoxyhemoglobin) within this MCA distribution infarct, identified due to the abnormal low signal intensity.

between brain with markedly reduced CBF (< 12 cm^3/100 g/min) in the irreversibly infarcted core and potentially salvageable brain tissue in areas where CBF is reduced (12-22 cm^3/100 g/min, with normal being ≈ 50) or MTT prolonged, the ischemic penumbra. Treatment options in the acute time period are in part dictated by the presence and extent of an ischemic penumbra (tissue at risk). CT perfusion also adds greatly to the detectability of early infarcts, with even small cortical lesions able to be diagnosed in two-thirds of cases. Whole brain pCT performs worst in the detection of very small (< 15 mm) lacunar infarcts, revealing only about one-fifth of these lesions. Without perfusion studies, acute infarcts (even very large lesions) can be difficult to detect on CT.

As evident by MR, few strokes demonstrate high signal intensity on FLAIR (which detects vasogenic edema well) within the first 4 hours. However, cell swelling (cytotoxic edema) develops within minutes following ischemia, leading to decreased ADC values

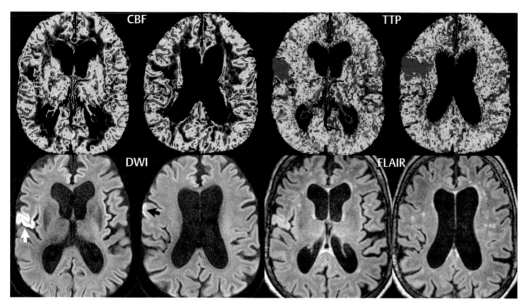

Fig. 4.5 Treatment of a small acute ischemic stroke with intravenous thrombolysis. CT was performed 1.5 hours following acute onset of hemiparesis, with intravenous recombinant tissue plasminogen activator (rtPA) given immediately thereafter. The CT was normal, other than the perfusion study (presented), which showed low CBV and CBF peripherally within a small portion of the MCA territory, with a slightly larger area of prolonged TTP. On MR, performed 24 hours later, restricted diffusion is present in the subcentral gyrus (*white arrow*), with only subtle changes in the precentral gyrus (*black arrow*). The FLAIR scan reveals scattered chronic small vessel ischemic changes, together with subtle abnormal high SI in the subcentral gyrus. The outcome in terms of involvement of the precentral gyrus is improved, as assessed by MR, most likely due to thrombolytic therapy.

and thus high signal intensity on DWI. MR is, on this basis (as well as other advantages), markedly more sensitive than CT for detection of early brain infarcts, with these being detected by DWI. In cytotoxic edema, there is impaired function of the sodium-potassium pump, leading to a net flow of water into the cell. There is no change in overall water content of the tissue. With MR, several scan sequences are typically acquired and compared, in addition to evaluation by more quantitative measures, specifically MR brain perfusion, in order to detect areas of "mismatch" and thus potential suitability for thrombolysis. This includes a comparison of FLAIR and DWI (identifying the area for which FLAIR is positive and DWI negative), and assessment of the mismatch between the area of diffusion restriction and the perfusion abnormality. A very small number (well less than 5%) of strokes are said to be initially DWI negative. This finding, published in the literature, was seen primarily with small lacunar infarcts and those in the brainstem, and likely reflects at least in part suboptimal imaging technique. On postcontrast T1-weighted exams, intravascular enhancement is occasionally seen in large acute territorial infarcts.

Digital subtraction angiography (DSA) may be subsequently obtained for either intra-arterial thrombolysis or mechanical thrombectomy. Major vessel occlusions are easily identified as vessel cutoffs. Collateral flow from pial-leptomeningeal anastomoses can also be visualized.

An important differential diagnosis in acute stroke triage, and indeed more generally for ischemia, is vasculitis. Imaging findings on DSA include vessel irregularities, stenoses, and occlusions in a pattern atypical for atherosclerosis. On MR, the most characteristic finding for vasculitis is that of multiple subcortical infarcts (**Fig. 4.8**). There is considerable variation, from patient to patient, in size, location, and number of lesions. Multiplanar, high-resolution, thin section, postcontrast, T1-weighted imaging depicts smooth, concentric arterial wall thickening and enhancement in

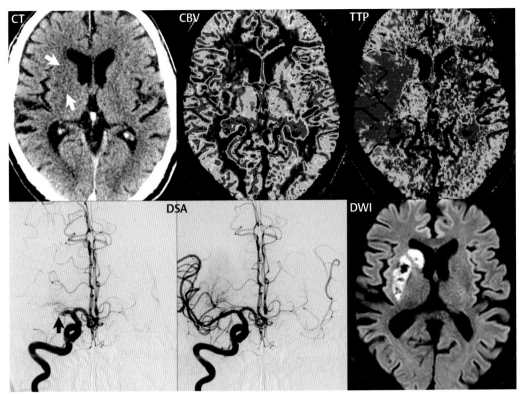

Fig. 4.6 Acute occlusion of the M1 segment of the MCA, with a mismatch between the infarct core and ischemic penumbra, treated using a stent retriever. At presentation on CT, there is subtle loss of definition of the right caudate and lentiform nuclei (*white arrows*). There is reduced CBV (*dark blue*) in the basal ganglia on the right, with a much larger ischemic penumbra (*red*) as defined by increased time to peak (TTP). DSA confirms the complete occlusion of the M1 segment (*black arrow*), with good collateral circulation through the ipsilateral ACA and PCA (images not shown). Following thrombectomy performed using a stent retriever, flow in the MCA is restored, with good visualization of peripheral branches (second DSA). The follow-up MR reveals restricted diffusion (and hemorrhage) within the basal ganglia, but without evidence of ischemia in the more distal MCA territory.

the majority of patients with cerebral vasculitis. However, intracranial arterial wall thickening and enhancement are also seen following mechanical thrombectomy, potentially mimicking the appearance of vasculitis on MR.

Brain death is occasionally imaged on CT, with characteristic findings including global brain swelling and ischemia (with loss of gray-white matter differentiation), an important appearance to know and thus readily recognize prospectively.

■ Subacute Cerebral Infarcts

The subacute time frame is generally defined as that from 24 to 48 hours after initial clinical

symptoms to 6 to 8 weeks. The subacute time period is sometimes subdivided into early subacute (first week) and late subacute (1 to 8 weeks in age) infarcts. This subdivision reflects in part that first week infarcts generally do not display blood-brain barrier disruption, whereas later subacute infarcts do, and thus, later infarcts typically display abnormal contrast enhancement on MR.

By 24 hours, vasogenic edema is present in 90% of brain infarcts, representing an overall increase in tissue water content. Vasogenic edema is seen with abnormal high signal intensity on T2-weighted scans and corresponding low signal intensity on T1-weighted scans, due to prolongation of both relaxation times. Vasogenic edema is seen as

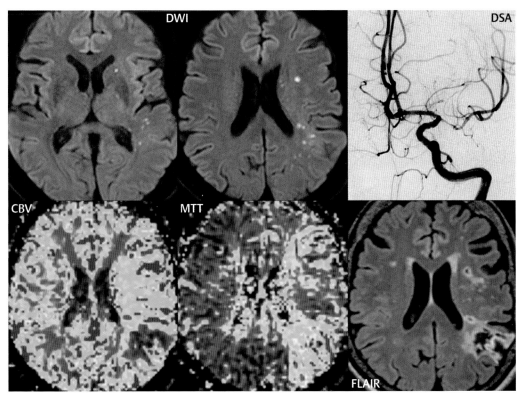

Fig. 4.7 Early ischemia in a patient not amenable to endovascular treatment, with temporal progression. The initial MR reveals multiple, small, punctate acute ischemic lesions (with high SI on DWI), predominantly in white matter and within the corona radiata. DSA shows a long segment of severe stenosis of the proximal M1 segment of the MCA, from which multiple small lenticulostriate branches arise, with endovascular treatment thus not recommended. TOF MRA also demonstrated this stenosis on the initial MR exam (not shown). A week after the initial MR, a perfusion MR (only) was obtained, with the CBV and MTT maps presented. In the parietal lobe, there is a large area with reduced CBV and prolonged MTT, representing a further progression of ischemic changes. The final follow-up, a FLAIR image, obtained 2 months later demonstrates extensive cystic encephalomalacia and gliosis in this region, consistent with a chronic infarct.

an area of low attenuation compared to normal adjacent brain on CT. Vasogenic edema persists for weeks. However, edema and mass effect typically peak in the middle of the first week, with necrosis and cavitation occurring subsequently.

Most thromboembolic strokes are initially nonhemorrhagic. Hemorrhagic transformation occurs in up to one-fourth of cases during the first week (**Fig. 4.9**). Due to ischemia, there is damage to the blood-brain barrier. When perfusion is reestablished, exudation of red blood cells causes parenchymal hemorrhage. Petechial hemorrhage is more common than a parenchymal hematoma. Cortical and basal ganglia hemorrhage are most common. Predisposing factors include lysis of an embolus,

opening of collaterals, restoration of normal blood pressure following hypotension, hypertension, and anticoagulation. Hemorrhage within an ischemic infarct is more commonly observed on MR than on CT, with MR more sensitive to blood products.

Large early subacute infarcts have prominent mass effect, with edema and mass effect subsiding by the late subacute time frame. Large infarcts (excluding lacunar infarcts) are commonly wedge-shaped, with involvement of both gray and white matter specifically in an arterial distribution. Blood-brain barrier disruption, as demonstrated by abnormal contrast enhancement, is common after 1 week and can be seen up to 6 to 8 weeks following stroke onset. However, blood-brain barrier

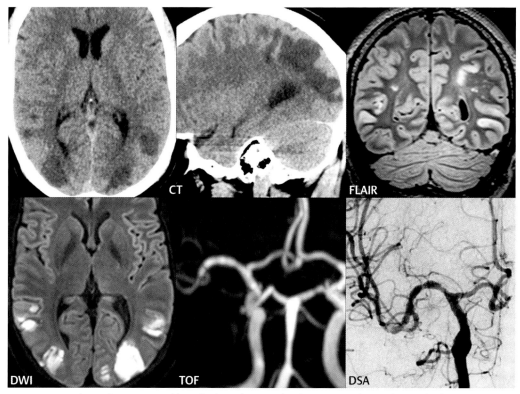

Fig. 4.8 Vasculitis. This 34-year-old multiple substance abuser presented with bilateral parietal infarcts, seen on both CT (axial and sagittal) and MR (coronal and axial), in a pattern consistent with vasculitis. TOF MRA revealed irregularity of the M1 segment of the MCA bilaterally (with the findings on the right shown), together with a marked stenosis involving the basilar artery. DSA was consistent with chronic vasculitis, demonstrating multiple proximal and more distal focal stenoses, with marked irregularity in vessel caliber (the involvement of the M1 segment of the right MCA is illustrated).

disruption can be seen as early as 2 days after clinical presentation.

On NECT, early infarcts may be isodense to normal brain and difficult to visualize, or may demonstrate subtle hypodensity. By 24 to 48 hours after presentation, most infarcts will be well identified with moderate hypodensity on CT (**Fig. 4.10**). Chronic infarcts appear as very hypodense, with a caveat being that an early subacute infarct can on occasion have this appearance. The presence or absence of local mass effect allows differentiation. After 1 to 2 weeks, in the late subacute time frame, infarcts commonly become isodense on CT ("fogging"). Abnormal parenchymal enhancement will usually be present at this time in the area of involvement, making confirmation of the infarct possible. Several weeks later, low density will again be seen in the area of the infarct, due to tissue cavitation.

On MR, subacute infarcts demonstrate abnormal low signal intensity on T1-weighted scans, due to the presence of vasogenic edema. Mass effect is also well demonstrated on such scans. Hemorrhage, when present in the form of methemoglobin, is seen as abnormal hyperintensity. On T2-weighted scans, vasogenic edema is seen as abnormal high signal intensity and is thus to some degree better depicted than on T1-weighted scans. This is particularly true for FLAIR scans. Sequence parameters are adjusted in FLAIR in order to suppress the signal intensity of CSF, making the abnormal hyperintensity due to vasogenic edema and gliosis easier to identify. A return to normal signal intensity on FLAIR in the region of the infarct in the late subacute time frame can occur, decreasing conspicuity of an infarct. However, this phenomenon is very uncommon, in distinction to the "fogging"

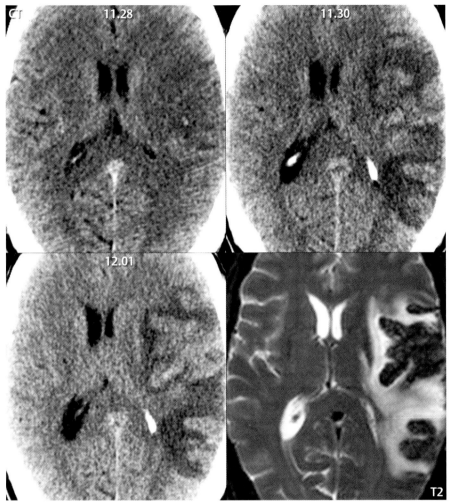

Fig. 4.9 Hemorrhagic transformation of an MCA territory infarct. At presentation, only subtle low density is noted in the left MCA territory. Two days later (11.30), an extensive infarct is noted with abnormal low density. However, there is also gyriform, mild high density within the involved region. One day later (12.01), this finding is much more evident. Note the prominent mass effect, with midline shift and compression of the left lateral ventricle. The MR was obtained a week later and shows extensive hemosiderin (low signal intensity) due to the petechial hemorrhagic transformation. The size of the infarct, the degree of mass effect, and the extensive hemorrhage are all prognostic of a poor clinical outcome.

effect on CT, which in published series is seen in the majority of patients. From personal experience, such infarcts are readily identifiable on postcontrast MR due to blood-brain barrier disruption. On T2-weighted scans (in particular those with T2* weighting, which includes GRE and SWI techniques), hemorrhage is commonly identified, with abnormal low signal intensity. The latter reflects the increased magnetic susceptibility of the blood component therein, with deoxyhemoglobin, intracellular methemoglobin, and hemosiderin all demonstrating this characteristic.

DWI plays only a limited role in subacute infarcts, in distinction to its critical role in the imaging of acute ischemia. Restricted diffusion, as reflected by hyperintensity on DWI and hypointensity on ADC maps, persists only up to 7 to 10 days. Once vasogenic edema is present, the abnormal hyperintensity on DWI has two contributions, that from restricted diffusion and that from the prolongation of

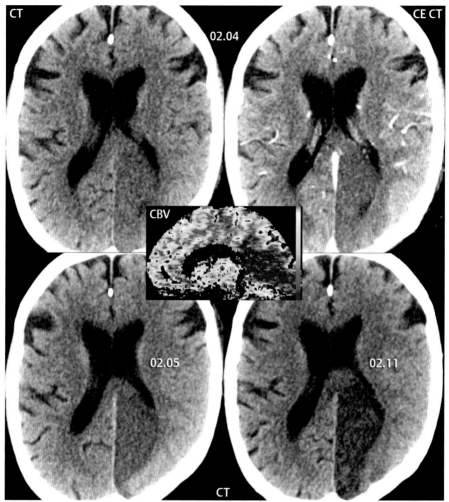

Fig. 4.10 Temporal progression on CT of a left PCA distribution infarct. On the initial scan (1 day after surgery, with the infarct having occurred due to a complication therein), precontrast, there is only subtle abnormal low density. Postcontrast, the abnormality is slightly more evident. The infarct is well identified, however, on the sagittal reformatted CBV image at presentation. One day later, the infarct is much better defined on the precontrast CT, with a progression in low density and mild mass effect. At 1 week following presentation, the infarct is very low density and has substantial mass effect upon the adjacent posterior left lateral ventricle. Although very low density is in general seen with chronic infarcts, it can also be present, as in this instance, in the subacute time frame.

T2. The former reflects cytotoxic edema and the latter vasogenic edema. After 10 days, subacute infarcts may still appear hyperintense on DWI. However, this is due to the phenomenon of "T2 shine through," with the signal intensity reflecting changes only in T2. This can be confirmed by the evaluation of the ADC map, which will not demonstrate restricted diffusion. After 10 days, and for up to several months, the ADC is generally increased in an infarct. Regarding the visualization of hemorrhage, DWI is usually acquired with echo planar technique, which has good sensitivity to susceptibility effects. DWI thus depicts well the presence of deoxyhemoglobin, intracellular methemoglobin, and/or hemosiderin. The abnormal low signal intensity due to the presence of these blood products can be seen on the b = 1000 diffusion weighted image, but is often more evident on the b – 0 image on which CSF is high signal intensity (the b value is the strength of the applied diffusion gradient, with b = 1000 the standard for DWI of the brain, and acquisition of an additional b = 0 scan required for calculation of the ADC map). The b = 0 scan can serve as a substitute for a T2*-weighted GRE image, if the latter has not been obtained (**Fig. 4.3**).

Time of flight MR angiography is often normal in the subacute time frame, even in large territorial infarcts. Vessel occlusion and/or stenoses can be seen but are not common findings on MR studies, other than those obtained very early following clinical presentation.

The patterns of abnormal contrast enhancement in brain infarcts on MR are well described in the literature. Intravascular enhancement reflects slow arterial flow and is the earliest type of abnormal enhancement seen. Intravascular enhancement can be seen on the first day and up to a week following presentation. A short segment of a single vessel or of multiple enhancing vessels may be seen. Meningeal enhancement, overlying the area of infarction, is the least common form

of abnormal contrast enhancement and is seen from days 1 to 3. These two patterns of enhancement have been described for large MCA and PCA territory infarcts. As previously noted, parenchymal enhancement, which is due to blood-brain barrier disruption, is common during the first month (**Fig. 4.11**).

As might be expected, there is considerable variation in the timing of parenchymal enhancement, which is usually not seen in the first few days and often not until 1 week. Parenchymal enhancement may persist for up to 8 weeks on MR following presentation. Enhancement of territorial and lacunar infarcts in the subacute time frame is the norm for MR, and for territorial infarcts is gyriform in appearance. In large territorial infarcts, the area of abnormal contrast enhancement is often less than the extent of the infarct, as defined by abnormal high signal intensity on FLAIR. Abnormal enhancement on MR permits differentiation of subacute from chronic infarcts, together with the identification of subacute infarcts in the midst of chronic white matter ischemic changes. Parenchymal

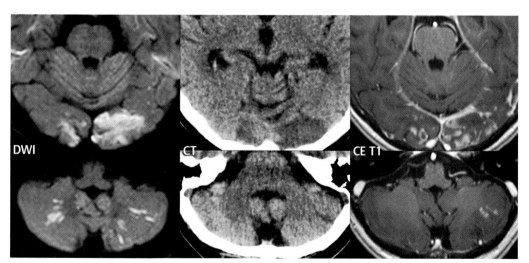

Fig. 4.11 Early subacute bilateral occipital and cerebellar infarcts, with temporal evolution to late subacute (enhancing) infarcts. MR (DWI) and CT obtained 1 day following major orthopedic surgery reveal bilateral posterior circulation infarcts (with restricted diffusion on DWI and low attenuation on CT, the latter corresponding to vasogenic edema). Note the relatively poor depiction of the cerebellar infarcts on CT, due to the lower intrinsic sensitivity to disease of this modality. An MR (CE T1) obtained 12 days later, in the late subacute time frame, reveals enhancement within a portion of the involved area of the occipital lobes and within some of the scattered watershed cerebellar infarcts. The patient was disoriented, with cortical blindness, at presentation. Visual field perimetry later confirmed partial visual field defects. The etiology in this instance was likely hypotension, in combination with significant atherosclerotic disease involving the posterior circulation.

enhancement can also be seen on CT, as previously noted, but is often less evident and is generally restricted to gyriform-like enhancement in territorial infarcts.

It is important to note one caveat in the differential diagnosis of subacute cerebral infarcts. If prior imaging is not available, a low-grade astrocytoma can be mistaken for a territorial infarct, in particular if it occurs in the PCA distribution (occipital lobe). This confusion is much less common for low-grade astrocytomas that occur in the MCA distribution. The reason for the difficulty in differentiation is that in the late subacute time frame there will be no diffusion restriction in an infarct and contrast enhancement may not be present. In addition, while the epicenter of a low-grade astrocytoma should be white matter, it may also include gray matter. Mass effect in the late subacute time frame will also typically be mild, as might be expected with a low-grade neoplasm. Close

image inspection to determine involvement of the cortex and to confirm that the extent of the lesion truly represents a portion of an arterial territory can prevent misdiagnosis. If there is any doubt, a follow-up exam at 3 months will provide definitive differentiation.

■ Chronic Cerebral Infarcts

The term *chronic* is typically used for infarcts greater than 1 to 2 months in age. With large chronic infarcts, findings include focal atrophy (volume loss), with widened sulci and ex vacuo ventricular dilatation. Both cystic encephalomalacia and gliosis are typically present. The former (cystic encephalomalacia) has CSF signal intensity on all pulse sequences, with the latter (gliosis) having high signal intensity on FLAIR and often noted surrounding the area of cystic change (**Fig. 4.12**). This distinction

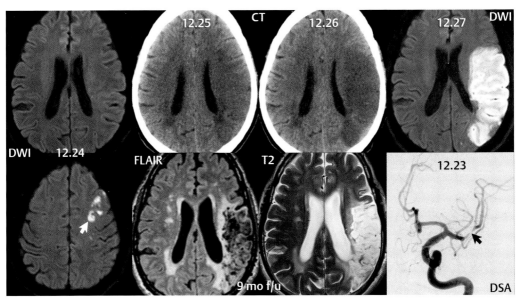

Fig. 4.12 Temporal evolution of a large left MCA infarct. DSA on 12.23 reveals a high-grade stenosis (*black arrow*) of the left MCA, distal to the origin of the lenticulostriate arteries, as well as the orbitofrontal and anterior temporal lobe branches. On the MR of 12.24, only a small acute anterior watershed infarct was noted (*white arrow*). By 12.25, on CT, subtle low density, effacement of sulci, and loss of gray-white matter differentiation are seen in the left MCA territory at the level of the lateral ventricles, reflecting a new large infarct. On the CT of 12.26, the infarct is much more evident, with lower attenuation. The infarct is also noted to include a portion of the watershed territory posteriorly. The appearance on the MR of 12.27 is similar, with a slight progression in mass effect. A follow-up MR exam obtained 9 months later reveals extensive cystic encephalomalacia within the area of the infarct (with CSF SI on FLAIR and the T2-weighted scan), together with gliosis at the medial, anterior, and posterior margins of the infarct.

and the identification of gliosis are more difficult on CT. In territorial infarcts, the area of involvement will be wedge-shaped, involving both gray and white matter. Dystrophic calcification, sometimes gyriform in pattern, can be seen in chronic infarcts on CT but is uncommon. Smaller cortical infarcts will have less prominent findings on MR and are often difficult to see prospectively on CT, with focal cortical atrophy and gliosis characteristic features (**Fig. 4.13**).

Wallerian degeneration, also known as anterograde degeneration, describes the degeneration that occurs involving axons distal to the site of injury. This is reflected by loss of tissue volume and, in some instances, by gliosis and thus abnormal high signal intensity on FLAIR (**Fig 4.14**, Parts 1 and 2). Wallerian degeneration is often seen in the corticospinal tract in patients with a large chronic infarct involving the motor cortex. Gliosis can be seen in continuity in the posterior limb of the internal capsule, the cerebral peduncle, the anterior pons, and extending into the medulla, where 80% of the fibers cross to the contralateral side.

The major differential diagnoses for a chronic infarct include a porencephalic cyst,

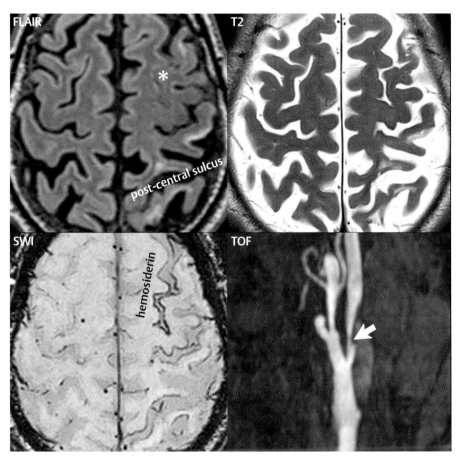

Fig. 4.13 Chronic cortical infarction (MCA territory). There is gliosis and volume loss involving the gray matter of the postcentral gyrus (anterior to the postcentral sulcus) and the superior parietal lobule (more posteriorly). Susceptibility weighted imaging reveals mild pial/cortical hemosiderin deposition, with abnormal low signal intensity. On the FLAIR scan, the superior frontal sulcus posteriorly on the left (*asterisk*) is isointense to brain, reflecting residua from prior hemorrhage. There is mild generalized cerebral atrophy. The MRA of the carotid arteries was performed with 3D TOF technique, as opposed to CE MRA, due to renal failure. There is a high-grade stenosis (*white arrow*) of the left internal carotid artery just subsequent to the bifurcation.

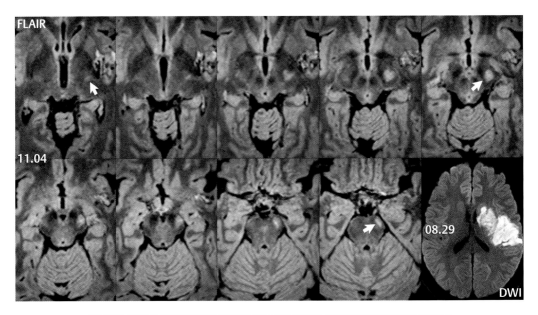

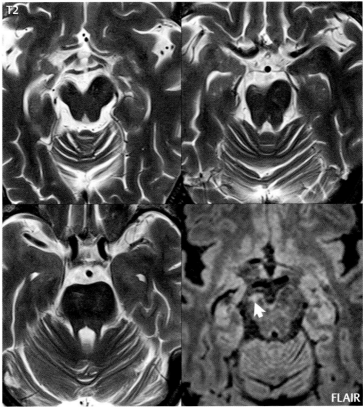

Fig. 4.14 Wallerian degeneration. (Part 1) A large left MCA distribution infarct, which includes the basal ganglia, is seen on the DWI scan (lower row, far right image) obtained in this patient at the time of initial symptoms (08.29). FLAIR images obtained 2 months later (11.04) reveal contiguous abnormal T2 high signal intensity extending from the posterior limb of the internal capsule (*arrow*), to the cerebral peduncle (*arrow*), and subsequently to the pons (*arrow*), within the corticospinal tract. Note that there is no associated atrophy. (Part 2) In a second patient, with a chronic right MCA distribution infarct, atrophy of the right cerebral peduncle and pons is seen on T2-weighted FSE images. There is minimal abnormal high signal intensity, corresponding to gliosis. The latter is best seen on FLAIR, with a small linear area of abnormal high signal intensity seen along the margin of the cerebral peduncle anteriorly (*arrow*).

posttraumatic encephalomalacia, and postsurgical changes. Identification of involvement of a vascular territory is critical in differential diagnosis.

■ Arterial Territory Infarcts

Infarcts in the major arterial territories are easily recognized due to their arterial distribution and their involvement of both gray and white matter. MCA infarcts are most common, followed by PCA infarcts. Of the three major arterial territories that encompass the cerebral hemispheres, ACA infarcts are by far the least common. As previously discussed, the MCA supplies the lateral cerebral hemispheres (including the insula and the anterior and lateral temporal lobes) (**Fig. 4.15**).

The lateral lenticulostriate arteries, arising from the M1 segment, supply the internal capsule, caudate nucleus, putamen, and globus pallidus (**Fig. 4.16**). The PCA can originate from the tip of the basilar artery (80%) or, in the case of a fetal origin (20%), directly from the internal carotid artery. The PCA supplies the posterior-inferior temporal lobe, medial parietal lobe, occipital lobe, and portions of the brainstem, thalamus, and posterior limb of the internal capsule (**Fig. 4.17**, Parts 1 and 2). Infarcts commonly involve only a portion of the entire arterial territory (**Fig. 4.18**; **Fig. 4.19**). The ACA supplies the anterior putamen, caudate head, anterior limb of the internal capsule, hypothalamus, corpus callosum, and medial surface of the cerebral hemisphere (**Fig. 4.20**). In rare instances, infarction can involve both the ACA and MCA territories (**Fig. 4.21**).

The posterior inferior cerebellar artery (PICA) arises from distal vertebral artery and supplies the retro-olivary (lateral) medulla, inferior vermis, tonsil, and posterior inferior portion of the cerebellar hemisphere (**Fig. 4.22**). The most frequent cause of a PICA infarct is thrombosis of the vertebral artery. The anterior inferior cerebellar artery (AICA) supplies a small portion of the cerebellum, anteriorly and inferiorly. Its territory is often referred to as being in equilibrium with PICA; specifically the larger the PICA territory, the

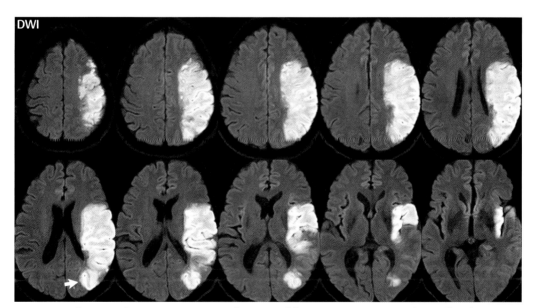

Fig. 4.15 Left MCA infarct, encompassing a large portion of the MCA territory. Multiple axial DWI sections are displayed illustrating the extent of this large left MCA distribution infarct. Note that the basal ganglia are spared, due to the arterial occlusion distal to their origin. The more anterior portion of the MCA territory is spared, as well as the majority of the temporal lobe, due to the occlusion occurring distal to the origins of the orbitofrontal and anterior temporal lobe branches. The infarct also includes a portion of the watershed distribution posteriorly (*white arrow*).

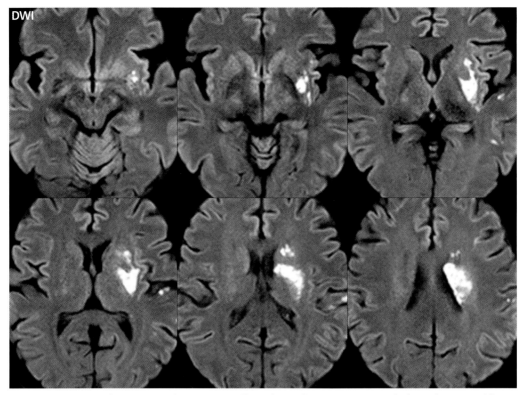

Fig. 4.16 Acute infarction involving principally the posterior putamen, external capsule, body of the caudate nucleus, and adjacent corona radiata. These areas are within the distribution of the lateral lenticulostriate arteries, which are longer and larger in diameter than their medial counterparts. This pattern of involvement is much less common than that involving the medial lenticulostriate arteries.

smaller is the AICA territory (and vice versa). The remaining arterial territory in the cerebellum is that of the superior cerebellar artery (SCA), which supplies the superior half of the cerebellum (and parts of the midbrain) and arises from the basilar artery just proximal to the posterior cerebral artery. The largest two cerebellar arterial territories are those of the PICA and SCA. Concerning territorial infarcts in the cerebellum, PICA is most common, followed by the SCA, with infarcts of AICA being uncommon. In the elderly, chronic small cerebellar infarcts are commonly detected on MR, often bilateral, and are seen in both major territories.

▦ Watershed Infarcts

Watershed infarcts occur at the junction between major vascular territories (**Fig. 4.23**). In the cerebral hemispheres, peripherally, there are two major cortical watershed zones. The first lies in the frontal cortex, at the interface between the ACA and MCA territories. The second lies in the parieto-occipital cortex, at the juncture of three arterial territories, the MCA, ACA, and PCA. These two watershed areas generally correspond anatomically to the posterior frontal lobe near the junction of the frontal and precentral sulci and the superior parietal lobule posterior to the postcentral sulcus. There is also a deep watershed zone (involving white matter), at the junction between brain supplied by penetrating branches (medullary white matter perforating arteries) and that by the major cerebral vessels (the MCA, PCA, and ACA) (**Fig. 4.24**). Involvement of this zone typically leads to a linear arc of ischemic tissue within deep white matter. Cerebellar watershed infarcts occur at the junction of the vascular territories for the three major vessels that supply the cerebellum.

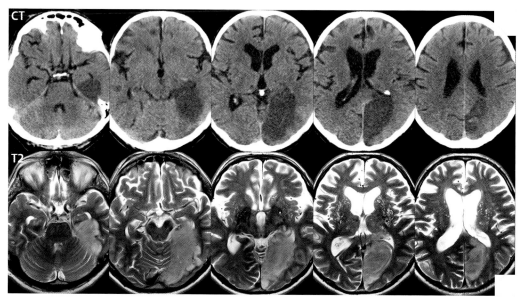

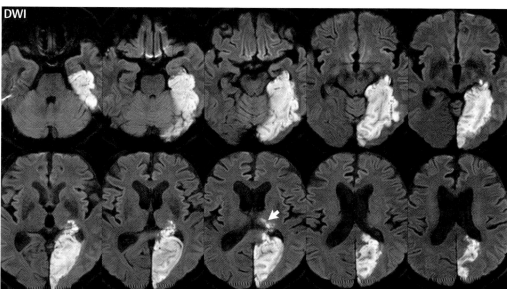

Fig. 4.17 Early subacute infarction involving the complete territory of the posterior cerebral artery (PCA). The patient presented after 2 days of dizziness with a right homonymous hemianopsia on clinical exam. The CT and MR (Part 1) reveal vasogenic edema in the medial, posteroinferior temporal lobe, the medial parietal lobe, and the occipital lobe on the left. There is mild local mass effect, with compression of the atrium of the left lateral ventricle, together with obliteration of sulci, the latter best appreciated on the T2-weighted scan. A portion of the thalamus also falls within the PCA territory and is commonly also involved, as in this case (*white arrow*, Part 2, DWI). Note that the thalamic involvement is poorly delineated on the T2-weighted scan and on the CT, the former due to the lower detectability of edema on this pulse sequence (compared to FLAIR, or DWI—which depicts the cytotoxic edema also present in this instance) and the latter due to the intrinsic lower sensitivity of this modality. Incidentally noted on the CT is a very small, round chronic infarct in the right thalamus.

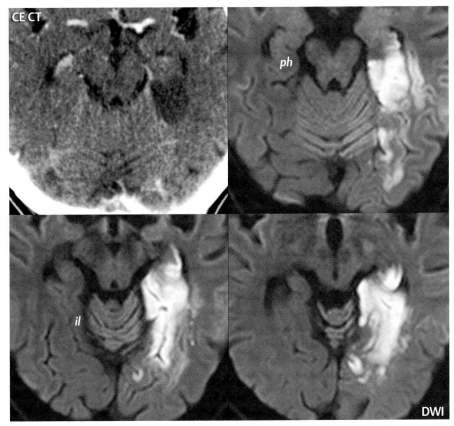

Fig. 4.18 Acute infarction involving a portion of the left PCA territory, specifically sparing the occipital distribution therein. Low density reflecting vasogenic edema is noted in the posterior medial left temporal lobe on the contrast-enhanced CT. Three axial sections are presented from the MR obtained the next day, better depicting the extent of the infarct (on the basis of restricted diffusion, due to cytotoxic edema) and its involvement of gyri. The infarct predominantly involves the parahippocampal (*ph*) and inferior lingual (*il*) gyri. Note also the involvement of the head of the hippocampus, along the medial wall of the tip of the temporal horn.

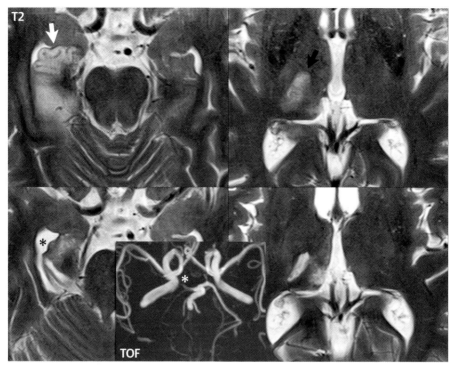

Fig. 4.19 PCA distribution infarct, involving the medial temporal lobe and thalamus, with temporal evolution also illustrated. T2-weighted scans are presented from 2 days following onset of symptoms (upper row) and on long-term follow-up at 18 months (lower row). By the time of the initial MR, vasogenic edema with abnormal high signal intensity is seen within both the hippocampus (*white arrow*) and the medial temporal lobe, and also in the thalamus (*black arrow*). At the time of this exam, there was also nonvisualization of the right PCA immediately following its origin (*white asterisk*) on the TOF exam (*insert*). On the initial follow-up MR (not shown), at 3 weeks after clinical presentation, flow was again present in the right PCA. On long-term follow-up, there is atrophy of the hippocampus reflected by ex vacuo dilatation of the tip of the right temple horn (*black asterisk*), with abnormal high signal intensity in both the medial temporal lobe and thalamus, reflecting a combination of gliosis more peripherally and fluid more centrally (better delineated on FLAIR, not shown). There is loss of brain substance in both regions. Note the involvement of two separate parts of the thalamus, both more laterally and medially (adjacent to the third ventricle).

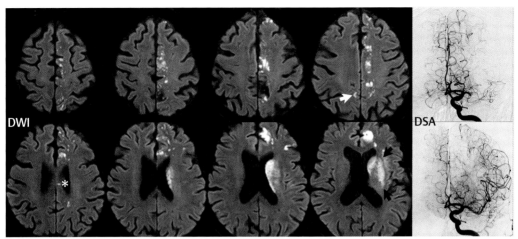

Fig. 4.20 Anterior cerebral artery (ACA) infarction, acute. There are scattered predominantly punctate areas of restricted diffusion (high SI) on the DWI images presented throughout nearly the entire territory of the anterior cerebral artery on the left. Only the corpus callosum is predominately preserved, although a small pinpoint lesion is seen therein (*asterisk*) on one image. Note the preservation of brain along the midline strip posteriorly, specifically on the more caudal sections, which represents the PCA territory. There is a very small lesion (*white arrow*) as well within the right ACA territory. The infarct involving the basal ganglia on the left (*black arrows*) preceded that temporally in the ACA distribution, with mild mass effect noted on the adjacent lateral ventricle. The ACA infarct resulted from fragmentation of an acute thrombus being removed endovascularly from the M1 segment of the MCA, with subsequent occlusion of the A2 segment of the left ACA. The initial DSA (top row) shows the occlusion of the left MCA, with good filling of the ACA and its branches on the left. The DSA at the end of the procedure (bottom row) demonstrates minimal recanalization of the left ACA with continued occlusion of many of its branches distal to the A2 segment (despite the successful thrombectomy involving the MCA).

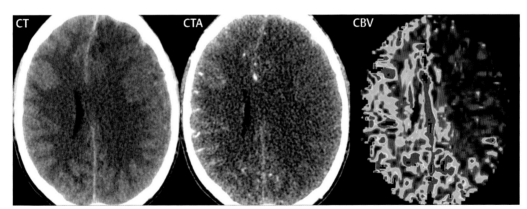

Fig. 4.21 Acute combined ACA and MCA infarction. There is left-to-right midline shift and compression of the left lateral ventricle on the unenhanced CT. Anteriorly, along the midline on the left, there is abnormal low density, consistent with an early ACA territory infarct. There is nonvisualization of the ACA and MCA branches on the left on the CTA. The CBV study reveals markedly reduced perfusion in both territories. If the ACOM and the PCOM on one side are not present, or otherwise involved (and not patent), occlusion of the internal carotid artery can cause ischemia in both the ACA and MCA territories. The etiology for ischemia in this 33-year-old patient was thrombosis of the ICA within the left cavernous sinus as a complication of sinusitis.

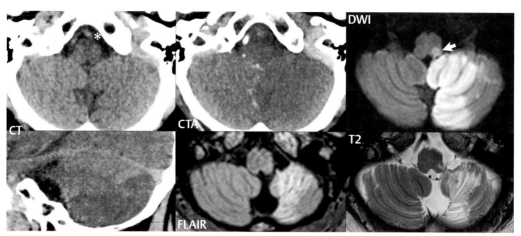

Fig. 4.22 Acute PICA infarct, with temporal evolution. The patient presented with dizziness and a severe headache. The unenhanced axial CT on clinical presentation is unremarkable. However, the CTA demonstrates thrombosis of the distal left vertebral artery. Note that this vessel (*asterisk*) is visualized on the unenhanced exam, but not opacified on the CTA. On the diffusion weighted MR scan obtained 12 hours following CT, abnormal high SI (confirmed to represent restricted diffusion on the ADC map, not shown) is noted in the left PICA distribution, primarily inferiorly, posteriorly, and medially. Note that the cerebellar tonsil, supplied by PICA, is also involved. A very small infarct is also seen within the posterolateral medulla (*white arrow*), a territory supplied by PICA as well. A thin strip of cerebellum is spared anteriorly, representing the vascular territory of AICA. On the sagittal reformat of the CT obtained at 24 hours, low density throughout the PICA territory is demonstrated. The FLAIR and T2-weighted axial MR scans obtained 4 months after clinical presentation reveal volume loss, gliosis (with abnormal high SI on FLAIR), and a small amount of cystic encephalomalacia (very high SI on T2, with lower SI on FLAIR) involving the left cerebellum. The small infarct within the medulla is also well visualized, with CSF SI (due to cavitation) on the T2-weighted scan.

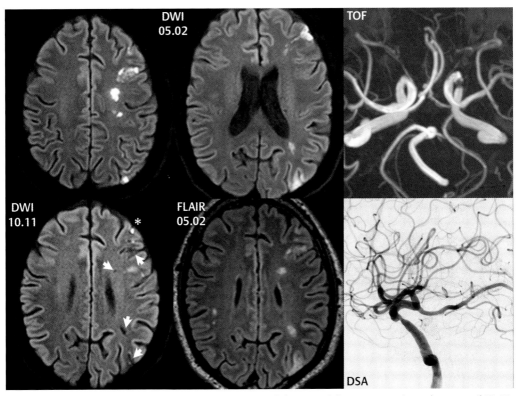

Fig. 4.23 Acute watershed infarcts, with two clinical presentations 5 months apart, due to a severe stenosis of the distal cavernous segment of the left internal carotid artery. Axial DWI sections at two different anatomic levels are presented from the exam of 05.02, revealing an extensive acute watershed infarct on the left. Note that the foci of abnormal high signal intensity form an arc, along the division between the ACA and MCA arterial territories on the first image and, on the second image, also involving posteriorly the watershed territory between the ACA, MCA, and PCA. The DWI image from the second acute presentation on 10.11 is difficult to compare to the initial exam due to a difference in tilt. The more posterior portion of this image matches the anatomy of the second, lower section from the exam of 05.02, while the more anterior portion matches that of the first, higher section. Multiple acute watershed infarcts were also seen on this exam, one of which (*asterisk*) is visualized on the presented image. By reformatting the isotropic high-resolution 3D FLAIR scan from 05.02 to match the plane of the 10.11 scan, the residua from the initial watershed infarct becomes clear, with small cystic regions and minimal associated volume loss (*white arrows*). Note that the small acute infarct (*asterisk*) visualized on the second exam lies immediately adjacent to a small cortical infarct seen on the first exam. Both the TOF MRA and subsequent DSA revealed the root cause—the severe focal stenosis of the distal left ICA.

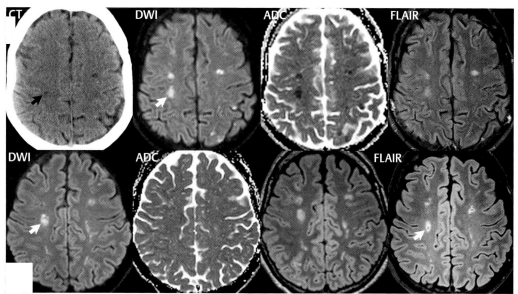

Fig. 4.24 Temporal evolution of small focal white matter infarcts (in a watershed distribution, due to a major hypotensive episode). The *arrows* point to the same lesion on four exams, the *black arrow* on the initial CT, the *white arrow* on the top row on the initial MR, the *white arrow* on the left on the lower row from the MR 10 days later, and the *white arrow* on the right on the lower row from the MR 3 months later. The top row depicts the CT and MR on clinical presentation, with multiple small white matter and cortical infarcts noted on DWI, only two of which can be identified on CT (illustrating the lower sensitivity of CT). The lesions have both cytotoxic edema (high SI on DWI with corresponding low SI on the ADC map) and vasogenic edema (high SI on FLAIR; however, note that the two lesions on the right side of the brain are just beginning to demonstrate vasogenic edema, being only slightly higher in SI than adjacent white matter). By the time of the second MR, the vasogenic edema of this lesion is more prominent, and there is no cytotoxic edema. Specifically, although the lesion is high SI on the DWI, there is no restricted diffusion (which would be seen as low SI on the ADC map), and thus the appearance on DWI reflects "T2 shine through." On the final follow-up (at 3 months), with a single FLAIR image presented, there is peripheral gliosis with cavitation centrally of this small lacunar infarct, the latter reflected by low signal intensity. The case also illustrates mild differences in the appearance of the brain due to differences in MR field strength and specific optimization of imaging technique (vendor). The initial MR was performed at 1.5 T, with the subsequent two exams at 3 T. The difference between the two FLAIR exams at 3 T (the two images in the lower row on the right) is attributable to differences in specific scan sequence parameters and acquisition software, both having been performed on state-of-the-art 3-T systems, but from two different major manufacturers.

Watershed infarcts are caused by hemodynamic compromise (**Fig. 4.25**). The maximum vulnerability to hypoperfusion occurs in the watershed zone. This terminal vascular distribution normally has a lower perfusion pressure. Hypotension, either with or without arterial occlusion or severe stenosis, leads to hemodynamic compromise. Blood flow in the affected watershed zone is critically lowered, leading to infarction. Symmetric peripheral watershed infarcts occurring both anteriorly and posteriorly typically reflect global hypoperfusion. Deep watershed infarcts are most often caused by regional hypoperfusion, for example ipsilateral carotid stenosis. In the presence of unilateral watershed infarcts, imaging is critical to determine whether a vascular stenosis is present and to assess its severity.

■ Multiple Embolic Infarcts

The presence of multiple small infarcts of the same time frame in several different vascular distributions is characteristic for emboli

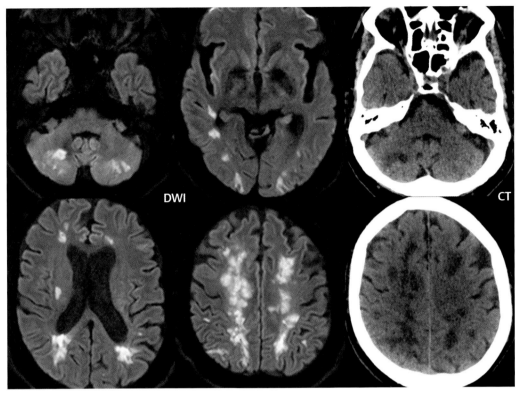

Fig. 4.25 Extensive watershed infarction. The patient experienced prolonged hypotension due to cardiogenic shock, with the CT and MR scans presented at 12 and 15 days, respectively, following that event. Selected DWI scans reveal extensive bilateral watershed infarction involving the cerebellum, the interface between the PCA and MCA territories in the occipital region, adjacent to the lateral ventricles both anteriorly (ACA-MCA watershed) and posteriorly (MCA-PCA watershed), and the centrum semiovale (ACA-MCA watershed). Although 15 days following the event, the infarcts still manifested some cytotoxic edema (with restricted diffusion). The CT is presented at two matching levels (that most caudal and that most cranial), demonstrating very low density consistent with recent infarction. Although not of importance for clinical management in this instance, the extent of involvement is better depicted by MR.

(**Fig. 4.26**). These can be cardiac or atheromatous in etiology. Cardiac emboli can be septic or aseptic and may originate from valvular vegetations, intracardiac masses (including specifically clot due to atrial fibrillation), or septal defects. Unilateral multiple small focal infarcts, in several vascular distributions (or simply within different parts of the MCA distribution), are most often due to emboli from atheromatous internal carotid artery plaques. Embolic infarcts often involve terminal cortical branches. Septic emboli are typically hemorrhagic and may demonstrate ring enhancement. In the differential diagnosis of multiple embolic infarcts is infarction due to a hypotensive episode (with hemodynamic compromise).

However, the latter typically involves watershed zones.

■ Lacunar Infarcts

Lacunar infarcts are small (usually < 15 mm), deep cerebral infarcts, most frequently seen with hypertension (**Fig. 4.27**). They result from occlusion of small penetrating arteries arising from the major cerebral arteries and most commonly involve the cerebral white matter, basal ganglia, thalamus, internal capsule, and brainstem (**Fig. 4.28**, Parts 1, 2, and 3). The small perforators involved are generally end arteries, with few collateral vessels. Lacunar infarcts are considered a hallmark

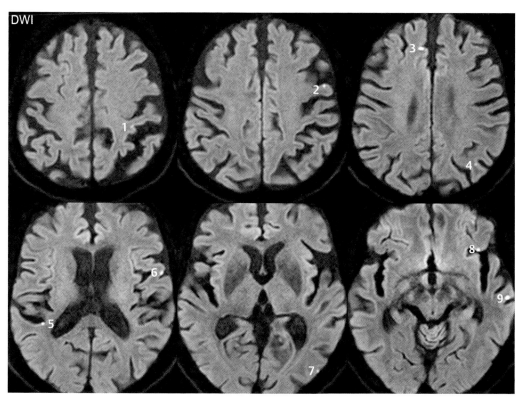

Fig. 4.26 Multiple punctate acute infarcts are noted on DWI, in a pattern consistent with emboli. The patient was an 87-year-old woman with risk factors for infarction including ventricular and supraventricular extrasystoles, hypertension, and diabetes mellitus. Infarcts are noted in the (*1*) postcentral, (*2*) precentral, (*3*) superior frontal, (*4*) angular, (*5*) superior temporal, (*6*) inferior frontal (pars opercularis), (*7*) middle occipital, (*8*) posterior orbital, and (*9*) middle temporal gyri.

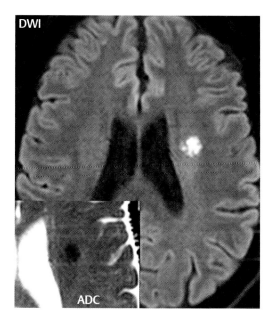

Fig 4.27 Acute lacunar infarct, corona radiata. A small, round, somewhat heterogeneous high signal intensity lesion is noted in the left corona radiata. Reference to the ADC map (*insert*) reveals this to be true restricted diffusion. The FLAIR scan (not shown) was also abnormal (with the lesion demonstrating high signal intensity), confirming the presence of both vasogenic and cytotoxic edema. The patient presented symptomatically 1 day prior to the MR, with the CT at that time normal.

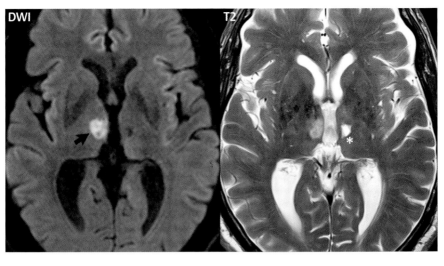

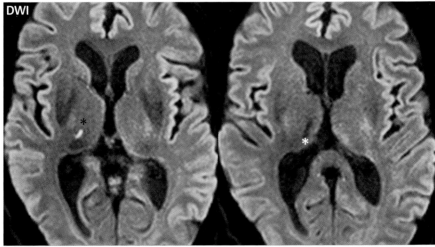

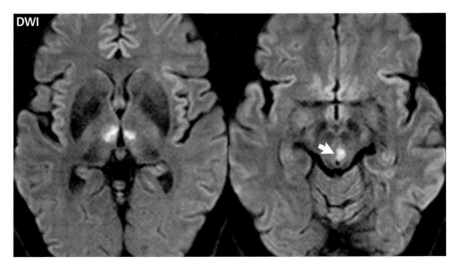

◀ **Fig 4.28** Acute thalamic infarction. Three patients with acute thalamic infarcts are illustrated. In the first patient (Part 1), there is a large acute medial right thalamic infarct (*black arrow*), with high SI on DWI (restricted diffusion), and a smaller chronic left thalamic infarct (*white asterisk*), with low SI on DWI and high SI on the T2-weighted fast spin echo scan, consistent with CSF. Bilateral thalamic infarcts are not uncommon and can easily be missed if the reader focuses on the initial finding only. In the second patient (Part 2), there is an acute lateral thalamic infarct (*black asterisk*) and a chronic more medial thalamic infarct

(*white asterisk*), both on the right side. In the third patient (Part 3), there are bilateral acute medial thalamic infarcts, with an additional medial brainstem infarct seen on a lower section (*white arrow*). The vascular supply to the thalamus is complex, with four major thalamic arteries supplying principally the ventroanterior (laterally), ventroposterior (laterally), posterior, and dorsomedial regions. Occlusion of the artery of Percheron, an anatomic variant in which a single dominant thalamoperforator from the P1 segment of the PCA supplies both paramedian thalami, results in characteristic acute bilateral thalamic infarction.

of small vessel (microvascular) disease. The clinical consequences of a lacunar stroke are highly variable and dependent upon location. Most lacunae visualized by imaging, particularly those in the cerebral white matter, are chronic and cannot be linked to a discrete clinical event in the patient's past.

On NECT, small acute lacunar infarcts are difficult to visualize. Old lacunae, however, appear as discrete focal CSF density lesions. MR is markedly superior to CT for detection of lacunar infarcts and, in particular, those involving the posterior fossa and brainstem. On MR, the acute and subacute time frame appearance is similar to that of larger infarcts, with restricted diffusion early and contrast enhancement in the late subacute time frame. Evaluating the temporal evolution of lacunar

infarcts on MR, cavitation and a decrease in size of the lesion with time are the norm. Chronic lacunar infarcts have CSF signal intensity on all imaging sequences. There is typically little associated gliosis. A just barely discernable hemosiderin rim is present in some instances. Multiple lacunar infarcts are often seen in the setting of chronic small vessel white matter ischemic disease. The major differential diagnosis for a cavitated chronic lacunar infarct is a dilated perivascular space.

In the chronic setting, it can be difficult to distinguish between the residua from a hemorrhagic lacunar infarct and a hematoma (**Fig. 4.29**). The latter often occur, in order of decreasing frequency, with hypertension in the basal ganglia, thalamus, pons, and cerebellar hemispheres.

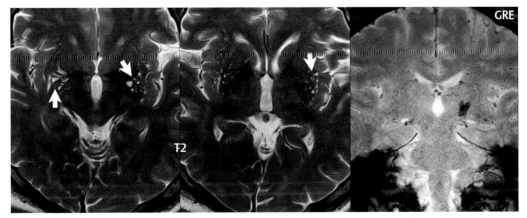

Fig. 4.29 Chronic, hemorrhagic, thalamic infarct in an elderly patient with dilated perivascular spaces. A small lesion is noted in the left thalamus, with low signal intensity on both the axial T2-weighted FSE (*black arrow*) and the coronal T2*-weighted GRE scans, consistent with hemosiderin. The lesion appears slightly larger and more prominent on the GRE scan, due to its greater sensitivity to magnetic susceptibility (T2*). Small cystic lesions (*white arrows*) along the distribution of the lenticulostriate arteries, particularly evident at the level of the anterior commissure (the first axial scan), simply represent prominent dilated perivascular spaces, a normal variant.

Brainstem Infarcts

Penetrating arteries (thalamoperforators) from the basilar tip and the proximal posterior cerebral artery supply the pons. Infarcts in the pons are most frequently unilateral, paramedian, and sharply marginated at the midline (**Fig. 4.30**, Parts 1 and 2). Bilateral pontine infarcts, which are less common, remain paramedian in distribution. Lateral pontine infarcts are uncommon. In the differential diagnosis for a unilateral pontine lesion is MS, whereas for bilateral central lesions, the differential diagnosis includes central pontine myelinolysis and pontine glioma.

In the medulla, both lateral and medial infarcts are seen. Lateral medullary infarcts, Wallenberg syndrome, present clinically with dysarthria, dysphagia, vertigo, nystagmus, ipsilateral Horner syndrome, and contralateral loss of pain and temperature sense over the body (**Fig. 4.31**). This is a known complication of chiropractic neck manipulation, due to dissection of the vertebral artery near the atlantoaxial joint. The arteries supplying the lateral medulla can originate from the distal vertebral artery or from PICA. Thus, a lateral medullary infarct can also be seen in a patient with a PICA infarct. Medial medullary infarction causes limb weakness on the contralateral side and hypoglossal nerve (XII) weakness on the ipsilateral side (with deviation of the tongue toward the infarct side) (**Fig. 4.32**). The blood supply is from the anterior spinal artery.

Gyral Localization of Cortical Infarcts

Accurate localization of small cortical infarcts, by the imaging physician interpreting the MR exam, can be extremely important to the referring clinician and clinical care. There are numerous atlases that serve as a reference for gyral labeling. These include the *Pocket Atlas of Sectional Anatomy, Volume I: Head and Neck, The Human Brain: Surface, Three-Dimensional Sectional Anatomy with MRI, and Blood Supply*, and *The Human Brain in 1969 Pieces*. In order to try to help the reader, numerous figures throughout this chapter are labeled in terms of the cortical gyri involved. This specific section focuses on more common infarct locations and identification of the gyri therein.

Turning first to the very basics, the central sulcus with the precentral gyrus anterior and the postcentral gyrus posterior is readily recognized and critical for localization of infarcts. This prominent landmark separates the frontal lobe anteriorly from the parietal lobe posteriorly, and thus the primary motor cortex anteriorly from the primary somatosensory cortex posteriorly. Representation of the different body parts in the primary motor cortex (as well as the primary somatosensory cortex) is described by the homunculus. The leg is represented close to the midline, folding along and lying within cortex at the vertex and along the upper portion bordering the falx. The lips, face, and hands are represented by an especially large area, which extends from lateral to more medial. A common misperception is that the map is clearly segregated; however, in reality, there is considerable overlap. The primary motor cortex does indeed contain a rough map of the body, but integrating muscles may also be an important part of its function. To localize the central sulcus on MR, it is important to first know that near the vertex along the midline in the frontal lobe is the superior frontal gyrus, bordered laterally by the middle frontal gyrus (**Fig. 4.33**).

The superior frontal sulcus is just lateral to the superior frontal gyrus and runs in an anterior posterior direction. It meets with the more superior portion of the precentral sulcus running left to right, to form an "L" (as viewed on the left side of the brain, and a backward "L" on the right). The sulcus immediately posterior therein is the central sulcus. The central sulcus is also distinctive due to the presence of a knob on the precentral gyrus, which corresponds to the motor hand area (**Fig. 4.34**). This general area is depicted in greater detail on multiple MR sections in a patient with an acute infarct localized to the precentral gyrus, but more specifically including the primary motor area laterally for the lips and tongue (**Fig. 4.35**).

The inferior frontal gyrus lies inferior to the middle frontal gyrus, with its posterior border

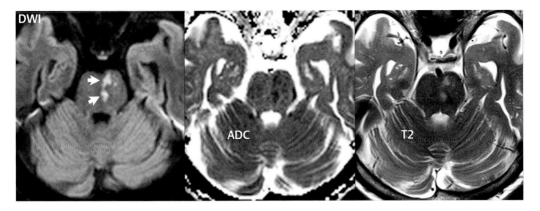

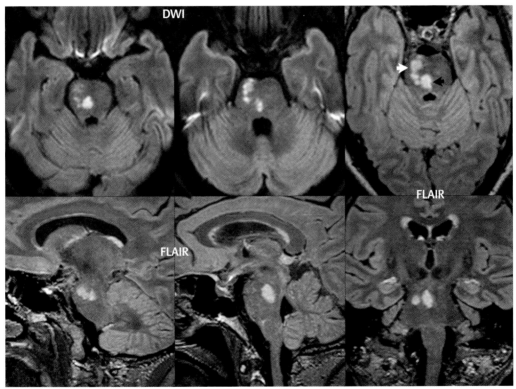

Fig. 4.30 Unilateral acute pontine infarct. In the first patient (Part 1), there is abnormal high SI (*arrows*) on DWI within the left pons, adjacent to the midline. There is corresponding restricted diffusion (low SI), consistent with cytotoxic edema, on the ADC map. It should be noted that ADC maps often have relatively poor image quality, being a calculated image, in comparison to the b = 1000 diffusion weighted scan, limiting assessment of true diffusion restriction in small lesions and also in areas often degraded by artifact, such as the brainstem. The FSE T2-weighted scan shows corresponding high signal intensity, representing vasogenic edema. In the second patient (Part 2), the infarct is on the right, having both a medial (sharply marginated along the midline) and a lateral component. Note that the more lateral component does *not* extend to the lateral border of the pons, which is characteristic. The axial and coronal FLAIR scans are thin MIPs from the high-resolution isotropic 3D data set, allowing both the medial (*black arrow*) and lateral (*white arrow*) components to be visualized on a single section. The sagittal FLAIR exam depicts, due to the different plane that they occur in, the lateral and medial components of this infarct on separate sections. The infarct in this second patient demonstrates, as in the first patient, both cytotoxic (with restricted diffusion on the ADC map, not shown) and vasogenic edema.

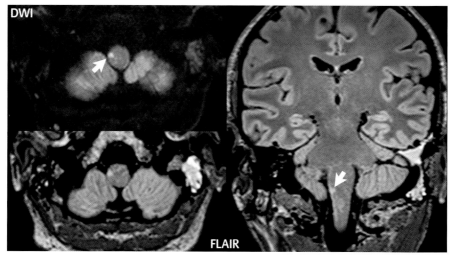

Fig. 4.31 Acute lateral medullary infarct. A very small area of hyperintensity on DWI (*arrow*, confirmed to represent restricted diffusion on the ADC map, not shown) together with high signal intensity on axial and coronal FLAIR images (vasogenic edema, *arrow*, on the coronal scan) is visualized in the right medulla. Careful image inspection is mandated for small infarcts within the medulla, which may only be visualized on a single image. This was the case in the example presented on the DWI, due to the 4-mm slice thickness, which is the current standard at 3 T. Detection and depiction of the lesion were improved by use of a high-resolution isotropic 3D FLAIR sequence, allowing submillimeter slice reformatted images in all planes. The patient was 40 years of age, with a history of hypertension and smoking.

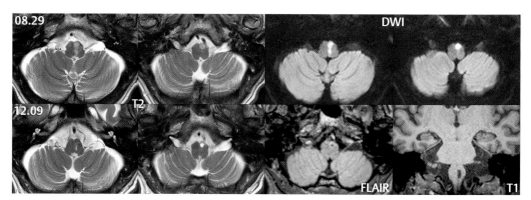

Fig. 4.32 Acute medial medullary infarct with temporal evolution. The patient awoke 2 days prior to the initial MR with right-sided paralysis. Two adjacent axial images through the medulla confirm a left paramedian infarct, with both vasogenic edema (high SI on the T2-weighted scan) and restricted diffusion (high SI on DWI, confirmed to be a true diffusion change on the ADC map, not shown). Follow-up MR 3.5 months later reveals mild gliosis within the lesion, with a small cystic area anteriorly (which on the FLAIR also demonstrates a thin rim of gliosis). The coronal thin section T1-weighted scan (from a 3D acquisition using MP-RAGE) illustrates the paramedian cavitated chronic appearance of the infarct in this patient.

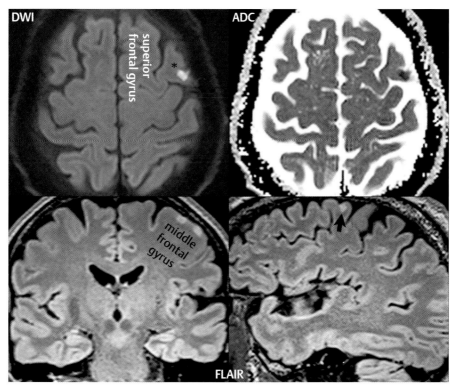

Fig. 4.33 Imaging of a small acute cortical infarct (*asterisk*), restricted to the middle frontal gyrus, in a 66-year-old man. The patient presented with anomic aphasia (difficulty in recalling words, names, and numbers) and problems with articulation, but no motor deficits. The superior frontal gyrus lies anteriorly and medially, composing about one-third of the frontal lobe (as does the middle frontal gyrus). Along its lateral border is the superior frontal sulcus, and then laterally lies the middle frontal gyrus. The other borders of the middle frontal gyrus are the precentral sulcus behind and the inferior frontal sulcus below (dividing it from the inferior frontal gyrus below). Isolated involvement of the middle frontal gyrus by an infarct, as illustrated, is uncommon.

being the more inferior portion of the precentral sulcus. Thus, it lies as well in front of the precentral gyrus (**Fig. 4.36**).

The insula is easy to recognize, being that portion of the cerebral cortex folded deep within the sylvian fissure. The latter separates in part the temporal lobe from the parietal and frontal lobes. The angular gyrus lies posteriorly in the parietal lobe, near the superior edge of the temporal lobe (**Fig. 4.37**). The angular gyrus is involved with the ability to write, language, and mathematics, among many other functions. On a sagittal view, it is easily identified by its horseshoe shape. The superior parietal and inferior parietal lobules lie immediately posterior to the postcentral sulcus. The superior parietal lobule extends medially to the midline, with the parieto-occipital fissure lying posteriorly. This lobule is involved in spatial orientation. The inferior parietal lobule is divided into two gyri, the supramarginal gyrus anteriorly and the angular gyrus posteriorly.

The terminology in the literature for temporal lobe gyri is somewhat inconsistent. Laterally, from superior to inferior, lie the superior, middle, and inferior temporal gyri. At the posterior end of the superior temporal gyrus lies the angular gyrus (**Fig. 4.38**). Inferiorly, and somewhat medially, lies the fusiform gyrus. Medially and superiorly, the lingual gyrus (posteriorly) and parahippocampal gyrus (anteriorly) together form the medial occipitotemporal gyrus. The uncus is the most anterior extent of the parahippocampal gyrus.

The occipital lobe anatomy is variable. Three gyri are generally described on the lateral

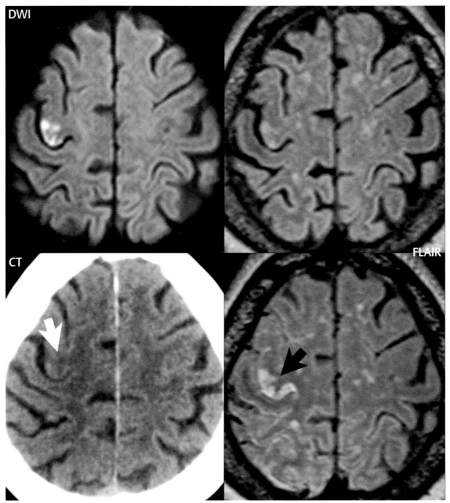

Fig. 4.34 Acute ischemia, the motor hand area. The first MR (upper row) is 24 hours following initial clinical symptoms (severe headache). Presentation to the hospital was at 16 hours, with the CT obtained at that time. The second MR (lower row, right hand image) was obtained at 42 hours following initial symptoms. Restricted diffusion (high SI on DWI) is seen on the first MR, accompanied by mild vasogenic edema (mild high SI on the FLAIR scan). By the time of the second MR, there is substantial progression in vasogenic edema (*black arrow*). Note also the more generalized mild inflammatory changes in the sulci of the right hemisphere and sulcal effacement on this scan. Despite the extensive chronic small vessel disease, the question of abnormal low density (*white arrow*) due to acute ischemia was raised on the initial CT. The lesion is within the precentral gyrus, but more specifically within a knob-like structure (along the "middle knee" of the central sulcus), shown by functional MRI studies to be the anatomic location of the motor hand area.

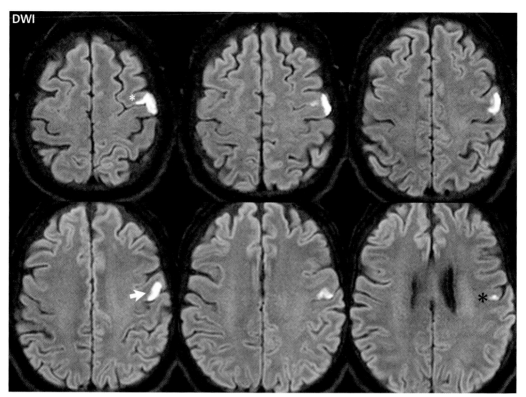

Fig. 4.35 Acute infarction restricted predominantly to the precentral gyrus (*arrow*), encompassing the more laterally located primary motor area for the lips and tongue (between the *arrow* and the *black asterisk*). The infarct extends superiorly to involve to a small degree the middle frontal gyrus (*white asterisk*). The patient presented with hypoesthesia of the lower lip and tongue on right, dysarthria, and deviation of tongue to the right. It should be noted that there is considerable variability between subjects in the location of primary motor and somatosensory cortex (traditionally being considered to be located in the precentral and postcentral gyri, respectively), with the localization of the two not divided in a simple manner by the central sulcus.

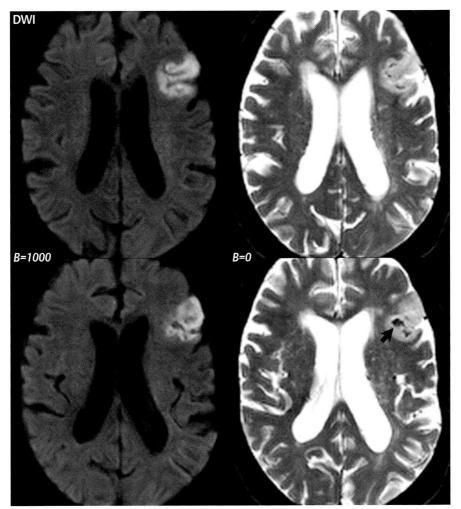

Fig. 4.36 Acute infarction, left frontal, inferior frontal gyrus. This 79-year-old presented with an expressive aphasia 1 day prior to the current exam. On the basis of a perfusion abnormality on CT at presentation (the scan was otherwise normal, specifically without evidence of hemorrhage), IV rtPA was administered. Due to patient motion, the MR scan was markedly degraded other than the DWI series. This case shows the value of DWI, both as a very fast scan (which thus may be diagnostic when other scan sequences are not) and also in providing a T2*-weighted scan (the b = 0 series). The latter can be used for the evaluation of vasogenic edema, which appears as abnormal high SI, and hemorrhage, which depending on stage can be visualized as abnormal low SI on T2*-weighted images, as with deoxyhemoglobin in this instance (*black arrow*). The area of involvement, the left inferior frontal gyrus, serves an important role in language production, corresponding to Broca's area.

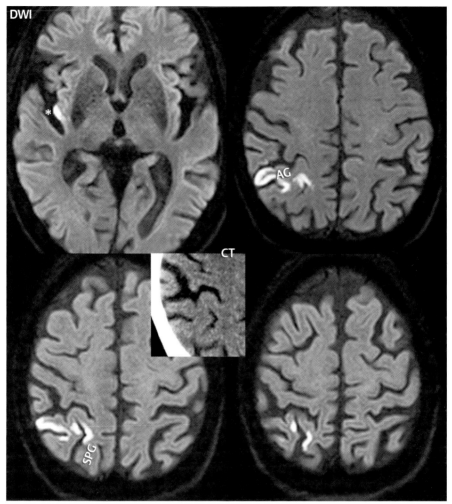

Fig. 4.37 Acute infarction involving the insula, angular gyrus (AG), and superior parietal gyrus (SPG). The patient presented with word-finding difficulties 2 days prior to the MR. The CT was normal at that time (*insert*), with specific comparison in retrospect of the involved regions. On MR, restricted diffusion is noted within portions of the cortex of the angular gyrus (with the supramarginal gyrus, just anterior and lateral, being normal) and the superior parietal gyrus (medially). A small segment of restricted diffusion is also noted within the cortex of the posterior insula (*asterisk*). Although the insula is within the MCA territory, the more posterior area of involvement is likely watershed in distribution and involves gyri that are less commonly associated with acute clinical presentations.

surface: the superior, middle, and inferior gyri. All three merge at the occipital pole. Medially lies the cuneus (Latin for "wedge"), a wedge- or triangular-shaped cortical area, bounded anteriorly by the parieto-occipital sulcus and inferiorly by the calcarine sulcus. Inferior to the calcarine sulcus lie the occipital pole and lingual gyrus (**Fig. 4.39**). The cuneus is a site for basic visual processing. The primary visual cortex is located in the occipital lobe, lying on both sides of the calcarine fissure.

■ Small Vessel Ischemic Disease

Patients with chronic small vessel white matter ischemic disease, an extremely common entity in the elderly patient population, demonstrate multiple, nonspecific, patchy foci of increased signal intensity on T2-weighted scans in the periventricular white matter, corona radiata, centrum semiovale, and subcortical white matter (**Fig. 4.40**). The involvement is usually relatively symmetric when

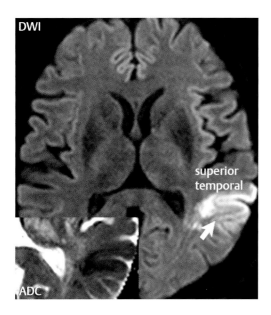

Fig. 4.38 Acute MCA distribution infarct, involving the angular (*arrow*) and superior temporal gyri. The CT at presentation, 20 hours prior to the MR, was negative; however, it did not include perfusion imaging. The ADC map (*insert*) confirms restricted diffusion, correlating to the hyperintensity noted on DWI. There was also hyperintensity in the region of involvement on FLAIR (not shown), corresponding to vasogenic edema.

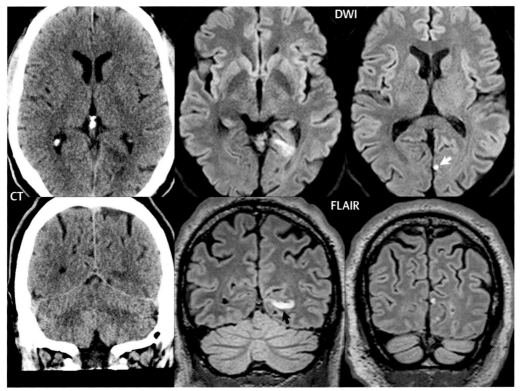

Fig. 4.39 Acute infarction in the left occipital lobe, presenting with a visual field defect. On axial and coronal unenhanced CT, a subtle low-density lesion is seen in the anterior occipital lobe on the left. Axial (upper row) and coronal (lower row) MRs are also illustrated. On MR, the infarct identified on CT is localized to be in the superior lingual gyrus (*black arrow*). In clinical studies, the lingual gyrus has been linked to processing vision. Also identified on MR is an additional pinpoint acute infarct (*white arrow*) in the cuneus, a small medially located region in the occipital lobe where visual processing of information from the contralateral inferior visual field occurs. The patient awoke in the morning with a hemianopsia. The CT was obtained at 9:00 PM that evening, with the MR 12 hours later. Both infarcts are shown on MR in the axial and coronal planes. The lesions are identified both on the basis of restricted diffusion (high SI on the DWI images) and vasogenic edema (high SI on FLAIR and low attenuation on CT).

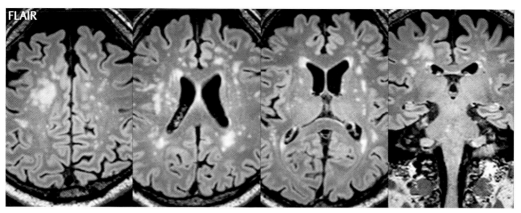

Fig. 4.40 Chronic small vessel white matter disease. There is patchy abnormal high signal intensity within the cerebral white matter bilaterally in this 72-year-old patient, well seen on FLAIR scans. These lesions represent the residua of ischemia and are common in atherosclerosis and hypertension. The presence of small vessel disease in such patients carries with it an increased risk of death and stroke.

comparing the right and left hemispheres. This disease process is also known by the term white matter hyperintensities (WMHs). The foci seen on MR correspond pathologically to areas of necrosis, small infarcts, demyelination, astroglia proliferation, and arteriolosclerosis. In long-standing advanced disease, the lesions may appear confluent. Progression with age is seen and, in personal experience, correlated with smoking; however, there are many possible etiologies and risk factors. A common rule of thumb is that one focal lesion per decade is considered to be within the range of normal. Thus, a few scattered FLAIR hyperintensities in the cerebral white matter of an older individual should raise little clinical concern. Confluence of the lesions adjacent to the frontal horns and atria of the lateral ventricles, in the periventricular white matter, is common in patients with advanced disease. CT poorly visualizes the disease process, although in advanced disease, there is often generalized, ill-defined, periventricular low density. On MR, FLAIR is the sequence of choice for best disease visualization. Chronic small vessel white matter ischemic disease is also poorly visualized on T1-weighted scans (as with NECT), a differentiating point on MR from multiple sclerosis. Chronic MS plaques are better visualized in comparison to chronic small vessel disease on T1-weighted scans due to the low signal intensity of the lesions relative to normal-appearing adjacent white matter.

■ Venous Infarcts

Venous infarcts can arise from dural sinus, cortical venous, or deep venous thrombosis. Superficial cerebral vein thrombosis can occur with or without accompanying dural sinus thrombosis (**Fig. 4.41**). Venous infarcts are somewhat distinctive due to their nonarterial distribution and frequency of associated hemorrhage. Vasogenic (as opposed to cytotoxic) edema predominates. On CT, a small vein, if thrombosed, may be visualized as hyperdense. The appearance on MR will depend on the specific blood product, but regardless, there will be absence of a normal flow void. 2D TOF and other MR angiographic techniques display the thrombus indirectly, by nonvisualization of the vein (and thus flow therein). With deep venous thrombosis, edema is typically noted in the thalamus, and the thrombosis may be unilateral or bilateral (within the internal cerebral veins), with the latter more common (**Fig. 4.42**).

The involved brain may demonstrate increased or decreased ADC values. Increased ADC indicates areas of impaired but viable

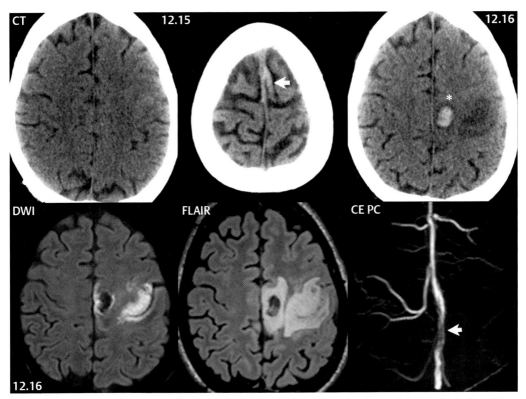

Fig. 4.41 Venous infarction with parenchymal hemorrhage. On the initial CT, a few gyri are not well visualized within the left frontal lobe (reflecting effacement), a subtle finding. On the axial section near the vertex, a hyperdense cortical vein (draining into the superior sagittal sinus) is visualized, suggesting clot therein. On the CT obtained the following day, the infarct itself is now directly visualized, with abnormal hypodensity, with an interval small parenchymal hematoma (*asterisk*) medially. DWI obtained the same day reveals both the hematoma medially, with abnormal hypodensity, and the cortical infarct laterally, with abnormal hyperintensity (restricted diffusion). There is extensive associated vasogenic edema, visualized on FLAIR as abnormal hyperintensity, both circumferential to the hemorrhage and associated with the venous infarction. The contrast-enhanced phase contrast venogram (axial thick MIP) reveals absence of a major cortical vein and its branches on the left, together with irregularity and narrowing of the midportion of the superior sagittal sinus (*arrow*), the latter reflecting additional clot therein.

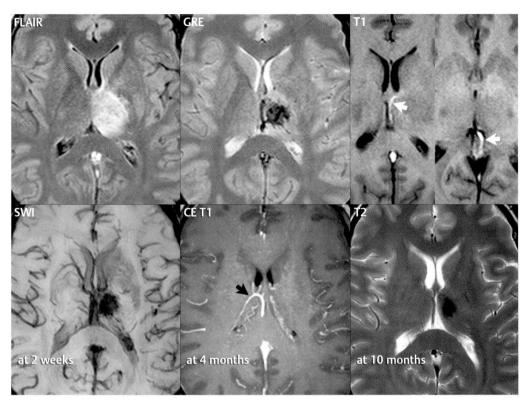

Fig. 4.42 Infarction of the left thalamus, due to unilateral deep venous thrombosis. On imaging, the patient presented with abnormal high signal intensity on the T2-weighted scan within the left thalamus, with mild mass effect, and no diffusion restriction (DWI not shown). Hemorrhage (deoxyhemoglobin) is seen within the lesion on the corresponding T2* GRE scan. Two axial precontrast T1-weighted scans reveal a methemoglobin clot (*white arrows*, with abnormal high signal intensity) within the internal cerebral vein on the left. A follow-up MR 2 weeks later shows the patent right internal cerebral vein as a flow void and the hemorrhage within the left thalamus as abnormal low signal intensity, on susceptibility weighted imaging (SWI). At 4 months, on a thin MIP of an axial postcontrast T1-weighted scan, the normal right thalamostriate vein (*black arrow*) is seen, draining into the internal cerebral vein, with these structures absent on the left (due to thrombosis). At 10 months, hemosiderin is seen within the left thalamus, as the residual of this hemorrhagic venous infarct, with no related mass effect. On this image, the patent right internal cerebral vein is also identified as a flow void.

tissue, with these regions free of sequelae on follow-up MR (with resolution of the thrombosis). If the ADC values are decreased, even strongly, it is possible that a complete recovery can be made, with a return to normal, but permanent neurologic injury can also occur. Areas of vasogenic edema that are nonhemorrhagic, with initially increased or normal ADC, have a good prognosis.

Less Common Presentations

There are several situations in which close image inspection is mandated due to the possibility of an infarct in addition to the primary identified lesion. Although the incidence of additional disease is low, without such attention, significant findings can easily be overlooked. One instance is the postoperative brain, following tumor resection. DWI images should be carefully evaluated for the possibility of a postsurgical infarct adjacent to the resection cavity (**Fig. 4.43**). Another instance is extension of an infarct, which can occur at any time following the initial presentation. This mandates evaluating carefully, in the case of

an infarct, the follow-up exam to exclude possible interval lesions (**Fig. 4.44**).

Complications following extensive vascular surgery, with stent grafts, can lead to an unusual imaging presentation (**Fig. 4.45**). The distribution of the resultant infarcts depends on many factors, including in particular collateralization via the circle of Willis.

Other Disease Entities That Feature or Mimic Ischemia

Sickle Cell Disease

There is a high incidence of infarcts in patients with sickle cell disease, with these commonly watershed in distribution. Clinically silent lesions, ischemic in etiology, are seen in deep white matter, with the MR appearance consistent with gliosis.

Systemic Lupus Erythematosus (SLE)

SLE is a multisystem autoimmune disease characterized by vasculitis, with CNS disease seen in 40% of patients. The most common imaging

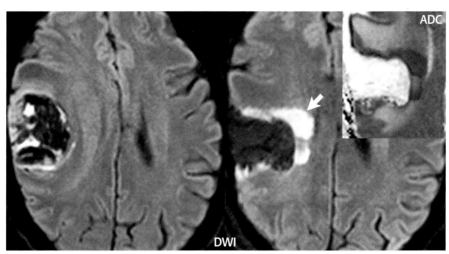

Fig. 4.43 Acute infarction, adjacent to the operative site, following resection of a glioblastoma. DWI scans are presented prior to and following resection of the bulk of a hemorrhagic parenchymal mass, which proved to be a glioblastoma multiforme (GBM). On the postoperative scan, a thick band of abnormal high signal intensity (*arrow*) is noted medial and anterior to the resection site, which is confirmed on the ADC map (*insert*) to represent restricted diffusion. Infarction adjacent to a resection is an uncommon but known complication, mandating acquisition and close evaluation of diffusion weighted scans following tumor surgery.

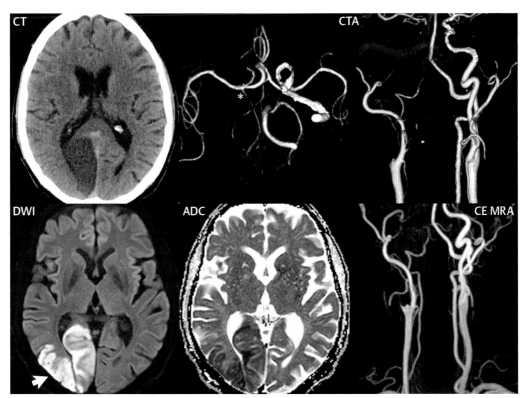

Fig. 4.44 Extension of an acute infarct. This 63-year-old man presented 1 day prior to the CT with homonymous hemianopsia. There is a clearly demarcated region of hypodensity in the medial right occipital lobe, with mild local mass effect (with both effacement of sulci and mild compression of the adjacent occipital horn). On occasion, as illustrated in this patient, an acute infarct on CT can be very low density, with distinction from a chronic infarct possible by the assessment of mass effect. CTA reveals a fetal origin to the right PCA, the latter being very small in caliber. There is complete occlusion of the right ICA at the bifurcation, atherosclerotic in nature. The MR was obtained 6 days later and reveals extension of the infarct laterally to include the watershed territory between the PCA and MCA distributions (*arrow*). Note that the infarct still manifests cytotoxic edema (with restricted diffusion on the ADC map), although this is more prominent laterally in the more recent area of involvement. The occlusion of the right ICA is again demonstrated, and appears similar on CE MRA to that on the prior CTA.

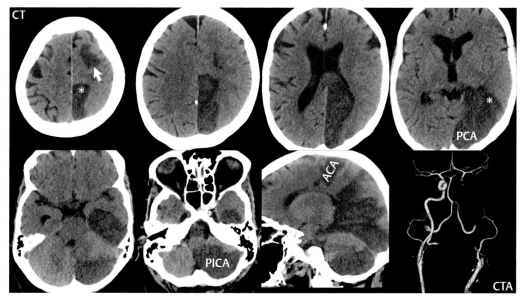

Fig. 4.45 Involvement of multiple arterial territories by ischemia in a patient following resection of a large thymoma requiring aortic reconstruction with several arterial stent grafts. On the CT obtained 8 days following surgery, low density consistent with infarction is noted on the left to involve a small portion of the ACA distribution (*arrow*, superior frontal gyrus) and the majority of the PCA and PICA distributions. The area of infarction includes a portion of the watershed territories (*asterisk*) with the ACA superiorly and the MCA laterally. CTA also reveals occlusion of the left internal carotid artery, with collateral flow via the anterior circulation sparing the left MCA distribution.

finding in the brain is that of multiple small subcortical and deep white matter lesions, which are hyperintense on FLAIR. As with most brain parenchymal disease, CT is relatively insensitive, with MR the imaging exam of choice. Discrete infarcts are less common but occur, and scans may reflect either an acute presentation or simply the chronic residual of such an infarct. Volume loss, focal or generalized, is seen long term in SLE. The differential diagnosis, strictly on an imaging basis, includes multiple sclerosis, chronic small vessel white matter ischemic disease, and other vasculitides.

Moyamoya Disease

In this disease, there is marked stenosis and/or occlusion of the terminal internal carotid arteries, together with the proximal anterior and middle cerebral artery branches. An extensive network of small collateral arterial vessels develops at the base of the brain, involving the lenticulostriate and thalamoperforating arteries (the "cloud of smoke" on angiography) (**Fig. 4.46**). Moyamoya is predominantly a disease of children, with an increased incidence in the Japanese and Korean populations, and relentless progression. MR reveals the multiple tiny collaterals, as flow voids, both in the basal ganglia and within enlarged CSF spaces. MRA and CTA reveal the narrowing of the supraclinoid internal carotid arteries and preferential vascular disease involving the anterior circulation. Collateral vessels from the external carotid artery may also be visualized. Multiple, bilateral hemispheric and deep white matter infarcts may be present, predominantly in the carotid distribution and in watershed regions. Surgical treatment of moyamoya includes both direct and indirect revascularization.

Tuberculosis

In tuberculosis, basilar exudates (meningitis) are more common than parenchymal lesions in the brain. Complications include communicating hydrocephalus due to blockage of CSF

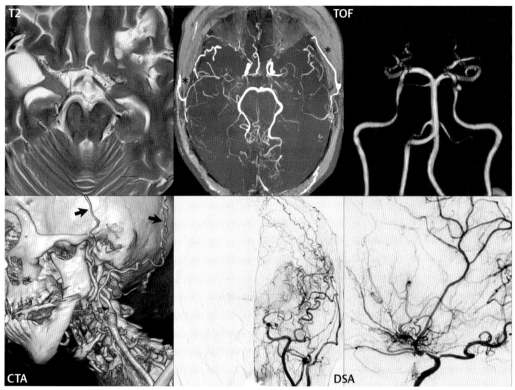

Fig. 4.46 Moyamoya, adult type, in a 51-year-old patient. Lenticulostriate collaterals are seen as a myriad of tiny filling defects within the suprasellar cistern bilaterally on the axial T2-weighted scan, with the proximal segments of the ACA and MCA atretic bilaterally. The thin MIP axial TOF MRA shows the distal portion of the internal carotid arteries to be small in caliber bilaterally, the occlusion of the MCA involving the M1 segment bilaterally, the prominent lenticulostriate collateral vessels, the small caliber of the peripheral MCA branches bilaterally, and the normal posterior circulation. Both superficial temporal to MCA branch surgical bypasses are patent (*asterisks*). The AP projection (VRT) from the circle of Willis TOF MRA reveals the rapid tapering and occlusion of the major anterior circulation branches, with the posterior circulation uninvolved. Functioning external to internal collaterals (*arrows*) are well seen on the CTA. A frontal projection from a left common carotid artery injection and a lateral projection from a right internal carotid artery injection are presented from the DSA study. The abrupt tapering of vessels, the prominent lenticulostriate arteries, and external to internal collateralization are well shown.

flow by the inflammatory exudate and infarction due to thrombosis of vessels coursing through the basal cisterns. Most commonly affected are the small penetrating arteries to the basal ganglia. MR is markedly superior to CT for disease detection and evaluation, in particular for basal meningitis.

Radiation Injury

Following radiation therapy, whether focal or whole brain, changes can be observed in the white matter on MR (but limited to the area of radiation). Vasogenic edema is seen early following treatment, due to damage to capillary endothelium, with limited clinical consequences. This finding is rarely seen on imaging, however, likely due to its low incidence and the timing of imaging exams relative to treatment. The late sequela of radiation therapy is that which is most often visualized and is due to axonal demyelination with increased water content. The imaging appearance of these late changes on MR is that of diffuse, symmetric white matter hyperintensity on T2-weighted scans, involving the periventricular white matter but sparing the compact fibers of the corpus callosum. The extent of involvement and specifically the degree with which more peripheral white matter is involved depend on many factors, including, in particular, radiation dose. The involvement of the white matter will be scalloped laterally, and in severe disease can extend to the cortical gray matter (but sparing the subcortical U-fibers). Radiation white matter changes are more common in elderly patients and with higher total radiation dose.

The time of onset from treatment varies. Changes can be seen within the first year following a single radiation treatment. Clinically, radiation white matter changes are most often seen in patients given palliative whole brain radiation for metastatic disease. In this population, the early changes can be somewhat subtle and restricted to the more immediate periventricular white matter. Commonly with time, this involvement will progress both in terms of the degree of abnormal high signal intensity on FLAIR and the extent of involvement of more peripheral white matter.

Acute Hypertensive Encephalopathy

This entity, also known by the term posterior reversible encephalopathy syndrome (PRES), is caused by acute severe hypertension. There is a predilection for involvement of the parieto-occipital regions (the posterior circulation), with bilateral, symmetric, abnormal high signal intensity (vasogenic edema) on FLAIR involving the cortex and subcortical white matter in a nonvascular distribution (**Fig. 4.47**). Involvement of the cerebral hemispheres may be more extensive in severe cases. Diffusion is usually not restricted. There may be accompanying involvement of the basal ganglia.

Carbon Monoxide Poisoning

Carbon monoxide (CO) inhalation results in impaired oxygen transport, with CO having 200 times the affinity for hemoglobin of oxygen. The hallmark of CO poisoning is symmetric injury to the globus pallidus. Initially vasogenic edema will be present, with mild

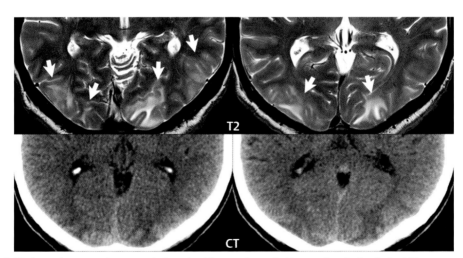

Fig. 4.47 Acute hypertensive encephalopathy. The patient presented with a severe headache, bilateral visual loss, and disorientation. There is abnormal hyperintensity (*white arrows*) on the T2-weighted scans in the parieto-occipital regions bilaterally, primarily subcortical in location but also involving the cortex. These findings would have been much more evident on FLAIR; however, the patient was combative and the FLAIR scans were markedly degraded by motion. Indeed, the MR requested the prior day could not be performed due to gross motion. Despite the use of a nonideal pulse sequence for evaluation, the MR is much more sensitive for detection of disease when compared to the CT. On the latter, regardless, abnormal low density can be detected in much of the involved area as depicted by MR. The follow-up MR obtained 1 month later was normal.

enlargement of the nuclei. With time, this is replaced by gliosis and cystic encephalomalacia, with the chronic appearance being one of symmetric atrophy of the nuclei. Pantothenate kinase-associated neurodegeneration (PKAN) can mimic the appearance of CO poisoning on CT and MR, with the term *eye of the tiger* used for the imaging presentation on T2-weighted scans and FLAIR. This progressive neurodegenerative disorder involves a mutation in the pantothenate kinase 2 gene, and today is classified within the category of neurodegeneration with brain iron accumulation (NBIA), of which PKAN is the most common type.

Osmotic Demyelination

This disease, previously referred to by the term central pontine myelinolysis, occurs due to too rapid correction of severe chronic hyponatremia (often in patients with alcoholism or malnutrition). In its classic presentation, there is abnormal symmetric involvement of the central pons, sparing the periphery, with high signal intensity on T2-weighted scans (which may lag behind clinical symptoms by 1 to 2 weeks) and restricted diffusion (seen early in the disease process). Extrapontine myelinolysis is most commonly seen in conjunction with central pontine myelinolysis (the term osmotic demyelination encompasses both entities), with symmetric involvement of the basal ganglia and cerebral white matter and, less commonly, other areas.

CADASIL

CADASIL (cerebral autosomal dominant arteriopathy with subcortical infarcts and leukoencephalopathy) is the most common hereditary stroke disorder. Patients present between the ages of 40 and 50 years with migraines, transient ischemic attacks, and strokes. The most common imaging presentation for CADASIL is that of multiple bilateral lesions involving the basal ganglia and white matter.

Mitochondrial Encephalomyopathy with Lactic Acidosis and Stroke-Like Episodes (MELAS)

This entity refers to a group of disorders that present with stroke-like symptoms. Presentation is most common in the second decade of life. Patients have in common deletions of mitochondrial DNA. The parietal and occipital cortex and subcortical white matter are most frequently involved, although any area of the brain may be affected. The imaging presentation is one of vasogenic edema, in involved regions, with subsequent resolution and development later of other regions of involvement. Lesions do not follow specific arterial distributions, a differentiating feature from thrombotic or embolic infarction.

Behçet's Disease

Behçet's disease is a rare, immune-mediated, systemic vasculitis involving small vessels. It is characterized by skin lesions, with CNS involvement in 25%, notably of the brainstem and in particular the cerebral peduncles.

Trauma

A cortical contusion is simply a bruise of the brain's surface. The inferior frontal and anterior/inferior temporal portions of these two lobes of the brain are particularly vulnerable. Contusions are well seen on FLAIR, with abnormal high signal intensity due to vasogenic edema. The characteristic location that these occur in and the fact that a vascular distribution is not involved, together with the clinical history, leave little confusion in terms of etiology. Hemorrhage is often also present. Diffuse axonal injury (DAI) (**Fig. 4.48**) and cortical contusion are the two most common findings with a closed head injury. In patients evaluated months to years following severe head trauma, encephalomalacia, with both gliosis and cystic changes, will be seen in areas of prior contusion. In severe injury, there may be resultant generalized cerebral atrophy.

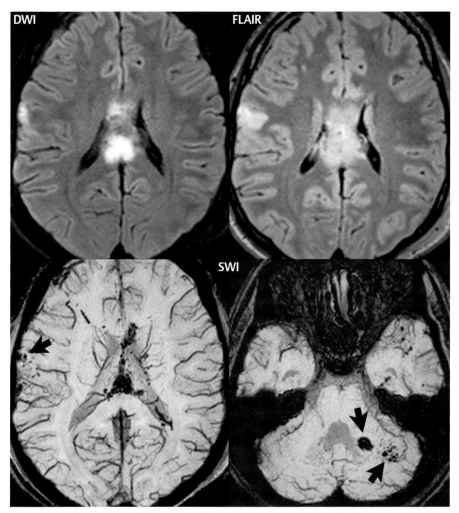

Fig. 4.48 Traumatic brain injury (diffuse axonal injury). The patient fell from a height, with CT (not shown) documenting several small parenchymal hemorrhages and a temporal bone fracture, together with a small amount of subarachnoid and intraventricular blood. The corpus callosum was normal, with CT having low sensitivity to traumatic brain lesions in general, and in particular those involving the corpus callosum. An MR was ordered due to delayed recovery of consciousness. Restricted diffusion (high SI) is noted on DWI in the corpus callosum on axial imaging (with corresponding findings on the ADC map, not shown), together with vasogenic edema (also high SI) seen on FLAIR. SWI demonstrates extensive hemorrhage along the midline within the corpus callosum, with low SI due to deoxyhemoglobin. Hemorrhage is also noted within the small, anterior parietal, cortical contusion and in the cerebellum (*black arrows*), the latter both in the middle cerebellar peduncle and more peripherally at the gray-white matter junction. Of these abnormalities, only that within the peduncle was noted on CT.

5 Aneurysms

■ Introduction

By definition, an aneurysm is an abnormal dilatation, typically saccular or fusiform in shape, of an artery. Intracranial aneurysms are thought to result from hemodynamic stress, abnormal remodeling, and inflammation. Saccular aneurysms are generally found at arterial branch points, although many are not clearly associated with branch vessels. Multiple lobes and daughter sacs ("Murphy's tit") are common in ruptured aneurysms. Rupture is typically at the apex. Although variable percentages in terms of sites of occurrence are published in the scientific literature, for unruptured aneurysms without subarachnoid hemorrhage, MCA, cavernous carotid (**Fig. 5.1**), and distal internal carotid are the most common (about 20% each), followed by PCOM and ACOM (including ACA) aneurysms (about 10% each). Posterior circulation aneurysms are least common, with about 5% vertebrobasilar/PCA and 5% basilar tip. The prevalence of aneurysms in the general population, without subarachnoid hemorrhage, is about 3%. The prevalence is higher in patients with atherosclerosis and also increases with age.

Multiple aneurysms are found in about 20% of all aneurysm cases (**Fig. 5.2**). Risk factors for multiple aneurysms include smoking and

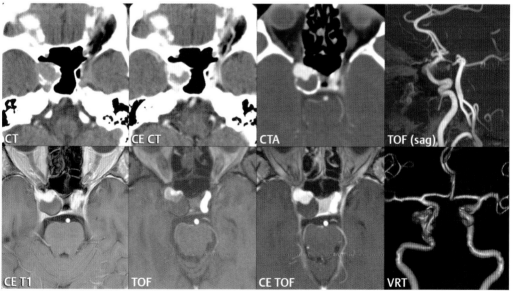

Fig. 5.1 Partially thrombosed, large cavernous carotid aneurysm. A round mass lesion is noted on the unenhanced CT within the right cavernous sinus. Postcontrast, there is enhancement of the anterior portion of the mass, with the imaging findings suggestive of an aneurysm of the cavernous portion of the distal internal carotid artery, with thrombosis of the posterior portion of the aneurysm. The CTA confirms this diagnosis, with the calcification of the wall of the aneurysm best depicted on this exam. On the TOF MRA, the patent portion of the aneurysm is poorly depicted, which is common with large aneurysms (due to flow dynamics). The patent portion is well visualized, however, on the additional axial contrast-enhanced T1-weighted image and contrast-enhanced TOF exam. VRT, with the view from anteriorly presented, shows the aneurysm and its continuity with the internal carotid artery well; however, inspection of additional rotations would be necessary to define the surface of the patent portion of the aneurysm.

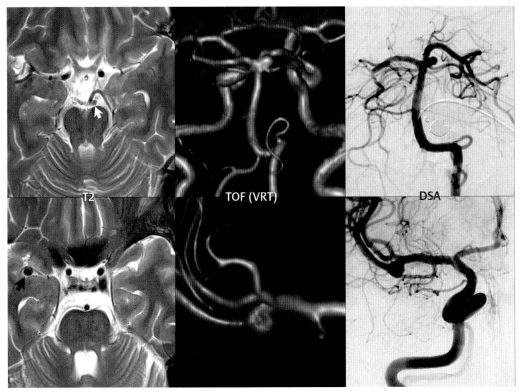

Fig. 5.2 Small unruptured aneurysms of the middle cerebral and basilar arteries. This case points to the importance of close inspection of high-resolution, thin section axial T2-weighted scans for detection of small aneurysms, and the critical role that TOF MRA plays both for detection and in depiction of brain aneurysms. The latter scan technique has markedly improved in recent years with routine imaging at 3 T and attention to setup (spatial resolution). In this instance, although the right MCA aneurysm is easily visualized (*black arrow*), as a flow void, on the axial screening T2-weighted exam, that involving the distal basilar artery (*white arrow*) is more subtle. Both are well depicted on the VRT images from the TOF MRA exam. The MCA bifurcation/trifurcation aneurysm arises at the origin of the inferior trunk, has a broad base, and incorporates the artery, measuring 7 mm in diameter. The second aneurysm arises from the distal basilar artery (but not its tip), has a diameter of 5.5 mm, is also sessile in shape, and incorporates the origin of the left superior cerebellar artery. Frontal views from the DSA exam are presented for comparison, with both aneurysms subsequently coiled.

hypertension (which are felt to be risk factors as well for development of a single, isolated aneurysm and subarachnoid hemorrhage). Infundibula, conical dilatations at an artery origin, are benign incidental findings not to be confused with an aneurysm. Intracranially, an infundibulum is most common at the PCOM origin.

There are several medical conditions well known to be associated with aneurysms. The two most important are polycystic kidney disease and a familial disposition. Estimates of prevalence of intracranial aneurysms in autosomal dominant polycystic kidney disease (ADPKD) range widely (up to 40%). The risk of aneurysm rupture with subarachnoid hemorrhage appears to be higher than in the general population, with presentation at a younger age. Twenty-five percent of patients with ADPKD and an aneurysm develop a second aneurysm within 15 years. Screening by noninvasive imaging is reasonable in ADPKD patients with a known aneurysm or prior subarachnoid hemorrhage or in patients who have a familial history.

In considering familial aneurysms, specifically when at least two first-degree relatives are affected, assessments of prevalence range widely, with 10% likely a reasonable estimate. There is a predilection for the middle cerebral artery, as well as for multiple aneurysms and subarachnoid hemorrhage at a younger age. Screening of such patients, if pursued, should be by noninvasive imaging. Other less common conditions with an increased incidence of intracranial aneurysms include Ehlers-Danlos syndrome type IV, α_1-antitrypsin deficiency, fibromuscular dysplasia, and in association with an arteriovenous malformation.

The natural history of unruptured intracranial aneurysms is controversial. The overall risk of rupture is likely 1 to 2% per year. The rate of rupture appears to be lower for small anterior circulation aneurysms. Larger aneurysms are at greater risk for rupture. However, if an aneurysm ruptures (with subarachnoid hemorrhage), the mortality rate is very high, greater than 50%.

Although a small saccular aneurysm may be visualized on a conventional MR or CT scan, 3D time of flight (TOF) MR angiography (MRA) and CT angiography (CTA) are specifically employed for detection and delineation (**Fig. 5.3**). CTA is the modality of choice in the acute presentation with subarachnoid hemorrhage, while 3D TOF MRA is often used for detection and evaluation of asymptomatic aneurysms, as well as for correlation and further definition of lesions in the acute setting and on follow-up. Modern scanners easily detect aneurysms as small as 2 mm in diameter. Treatment of intracranial brain aneurysms that have bled, or are deemed to present a significant risk to the patient because of potential bleeding in the future, is by either surgical clipping or endovascular occlusion. Surgery is much less

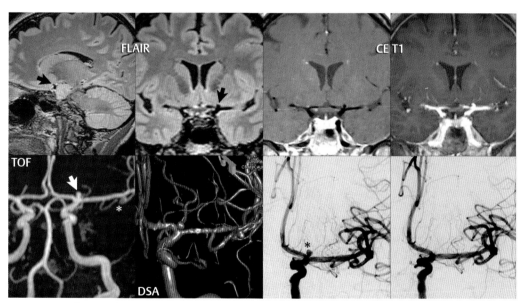

Fig. 5.3 Small carotid terminus aneurysm. Small aneurysms can be difficult to see on conventional planar MR images, further emphasizing the importance of TOF MRA. Sagittal and coronal thin section 3D FLAIR images reveal a small, low SI, round lesion (*black arrows*, corresponding to a flow void) just superior and contiguous to the terminus of the left internal carotid artery. On contrast-enhanced T1-weighted images, small aneurysms may either enhance or remain as a flow void, due to specific selection of imaging technique. On fast spin echo imaging, high-velocity flow generally is low signal intensity, while on 3D gradient echo–based techniques such as MP-RAGE, the vessels are enhanced.

Coronal images with both techniques, postcontrast, are illustrated in the upper right hand quadrant of the figure. A coronal thick MIP TOF MRA depicts well this small carotid terminus aneurysm (*white arrow*), also visualizing an additional MCA bifurcation aneurysm (*small white asterisk*). Twenty percent of intracranial aneurysms are multiple, thus mandating careful image inspection for a second (or third) aneurysm in all patients. The VRT image from DSA depicts well both aneurysms. Frontal projections from a left internal carotid artery injection are also presented, depicting the carotid terminus aneurysm prior to (*large black asterisk*) and following endovascular coiling.

common today, although not all aneurysms can be treated by an endovascular approach.

Aneurysm Treatment

Asymptomatic patients with untreated intradural aneurysms are followed in some centers by annual CTA or MRA. Growth or new symptoms, such as headaches or cranial nerve palsies, raise concern in regard to impending rupture. Cessation of smoking and appropriate management of hypertension are felt to be important. Treatment of unruptured aneurysms, if desired or indicated, is currently performed either by surgery or by endovascular means.

Surgical

Surgical treatment was considered in the past to be the gold standard for treatment (**Fig. 5.4**); however, complication rates are

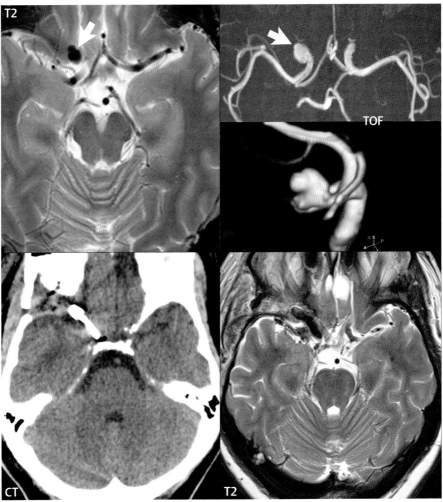

Fig. 5.4 Ophthalmic artery aneurysm. On an axial T2-weighted scan, an oval flow void (*arrow*) is seen in the vicinity of the ophthalmic artery. A thick section axial MIP of the TOF MRA confirms the lesion to be an aneurysm (*arrow*). The targeted VRT (from the TOF exam) demonstrates well the saccular, multilobulated character of this aneurysm, with the origin of the ophthalmic artery not incorporated into the sac (not shown well on the presented image). This aneurysm was surgically clipped, with the CT and MR (T2) following surgery presented. The surgical clip is depicted clearly, with little artifact on each exam, due both to improvements in CT technology and the use of metal alloys with decreased artifact (on both MR and CT). The changes in the anterior low frontal lobe are unrelated, due to prior trauma.

high. In surgical treatment of unruptured aneurysms, the mortality rate is about 3%, with permanent morbidity seen in up to 20%. Risk factors for surgery in this group of patients include age, size of the aneurysm (> 12 mm), and location in the posterior circulation. In surgical treatment of ruptured aneurysms, the mortality rate is about 15%, with substantial, permanent morbidity in an additional 15%.

In surgical series, the frequency of a residual aneurysm is 4 to 8%. Catheter angiography, which can be performed intraoperatively, is necessary to confirm complete occlusion of the aneurysm and preservation of associated vessels. There is an increased rate of rupture after clipping when a portion of the aneurysm remains, and enlargement of the residual portion of an aneurysm following clipping has been documented. Recurrence has also been shown in 1% of aneurysms after complete surgical obliteration, the latter confirmed by postoperative angiography (**Fig. 5.5**).

Endovascular

The complication rate with endovascular treatment of an unruptured brain aneurysm is approximately 10% (**Fig. 5.6**). The rate of permanent complications is less than half this figure. Repeat hemorrhage is uncommon, seen in 3%.

The advent of detachable coils, led by the development of the Guglielmi detachable coil (GDC) conceived serendipitously in the early 1980s, enabled development of the field of aneurysm coiling as we know it today. With this system, until the coil is in satisfactory position, it remains attached to the pusher wire. Detachment is achieved by application of a low-amplitude electrical current, causing electrolysis of the connection between the coil and the wire. Numerous technical refinements have followed, with an array of shapes and sizes available. Augmented (bioactive) coils continue to attract interest, with the goal to promote thrombosis and fibrosis, thus reducing the likelihood of subsequent

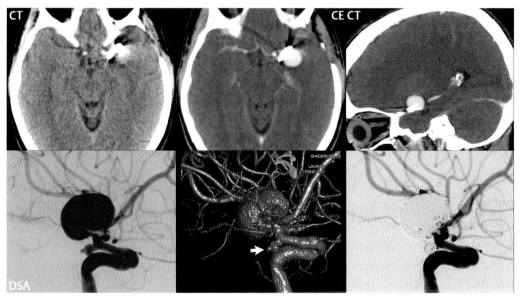

Fig. 5.5 Recurrent MCA aneurysm following surgical clipping. On the unenhanced CT, there is a question of a focal abnormal high-density lesion adjacent and just lateral to the surgical clip, placed 13 years earlier for a proximal MCA aneurysm. Postcontrast, a round 16-mm-diameter, enhancing lesion is noted, consistent with a recurrent aneurysm. No other aneurysms were noted on CT. A second aneurysm is identified on DSA, a 4-mm multilobulated aneurysm of the left posterior communicating artery. The latter is best depicted (*arrow*) on the volume-rendered projection. Both aneurysms were occluded with platinum microcoils, with DSA presented both prior to and following coiling.

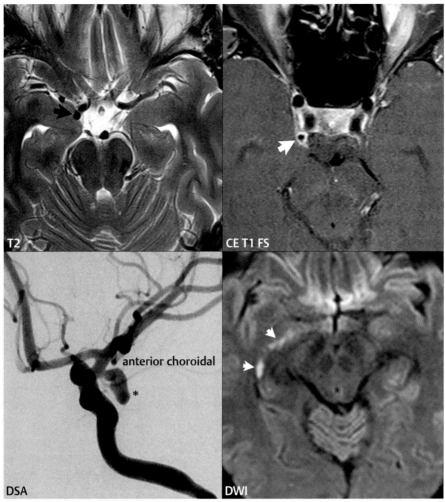

Fig. 5.6 Nonruptured aneurysm of the anterior choroidal artery. The patient presented with diplopia, anisocoria, and ptosis, due to compression of the oculomotor nerve on the right. A small aneurysm is noted projecting posteriorly from the internal carotid artery, seen as a flow void (*black arrow*) on the axial T2-weighted FSE image. Postcontrast, there is thin, smooth circumferential enhancement (*white arrow*), a finding seen in aneurysms on high-resolution imaging. On DSA, the aneurysm (*asterisk*) is confirmed to lie at the origin of the anterior choroidal artery (just proximal to the terminus of the internal carotid artery), being directed laterally and posteriorly. It has a narrow base and a maximum diameter of 8 mm. The aneurysm was subsequently coiled, with preservation of the anterior choroidal artery. On follow-up MR exam, obtained 6 days after coiling, a small infarct is noted (*small white arrows*, a known complication of coiling being thromboembolic stroke), with hyperintensity on DWI, within the right parahippocampal gyrus.

recanalization. Wide-neck aneurysms present an additional challenge, with one current approach being deployment of a thin wire mesh stent across the neck, within the parent vessel. Coils are then placed via a microcatheter that enters the aneurysm through the interstices of the stent, with the latter acting as a scaffold to hold the coils within the aneurysm. The relatively recent advent of flow-diverting stents, for example, the Pipeline Embolization device, may lead to a further paradigm shift in endovascular aneurysm treatment.

Complete occlusion of an aneurysm following coiling is reported in about 50%, with "near complete" in 90%. Recurrence after coiling (defined as recanalization sufficiently large to allow retreatment, either surgical or endovascular) is seen in about 20% of patients 1 to

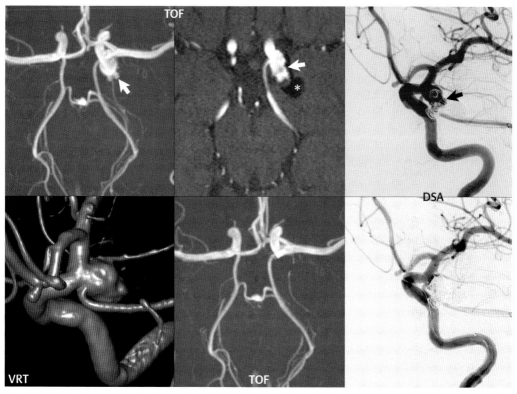

Fig. 5.7 Posterior communicating artery (PCOM) aneurysm recurrence following endovascular coiling. TOF MRA (axial MIP and source images) reveals a partially recanalized saccular aneurysm (*white arrow*), with a signal void in the coiled (nonpatent) portion of the aneurysm (*asterisk*). The subsequent DSA depicts well this recurrence (*black arrow*), with VRT demonstrating the complexity of the patent portion of the aneurysm, which incorporates the origin of the PCOM. Following re-embolization with platinum microcoils, complete occlusion was achieved, as demonstrated on both the follow-up TOF MRA and DSA. Aneurysm recurrence following endovascular coiling is seen in 20% of cases, whereas surgical series report aneurysm recurrence in only 1%.

2 years following initial treatment (**Fig. 5.7**). Larger aneurysms (> 10 mm) and those with a wide neck are more prone to recurrence. Recurrences are also more common following suboptimal initial endovascular treatment. In terms of the relationship to the parent vessel, terminal aneurysms tend to recur more frequently than sidewall aneurysms. Due predominantly to the risk of recurrence, long-term follow-up/surveillance with MR or DSA is recommended (**Fig. 5.8**).

Comparison of Surgery and Endovascular Treatment

Significantly lower rates of morbidity and mortality are found with coiling of unruptured intracranial aneurysms when compared to clipping. Decreased length of stay, hospital charges, and periprocedural complications also significantly favor coiling of unruptured aneurysms. With ruptured aneurysms, several studies have shown little difference between surgical and endovascular treatment, other than the greater recurrence rate following the latter. Other studies, and specifically the International Subarachnoid Aneurysm Trial (ISAT), have shown decreased mortality and significant morbidity in the endovascular group, together with a significantly reduced risk of vasospasm and ischemic neurologic deficits.

Flow Diversion

The concept of flow diversion involves placement of a wire mesh stent within the lumen

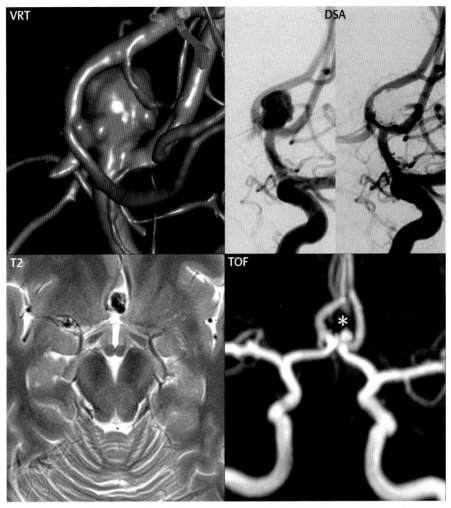

Fig. 5.8 Recanalization of a previously coiled ACOM aneurysm. The patient presented with acute subarachnoid blood on CT (not shown), consistent with a ruptured aneurysm. DSA revealed a complex, broad-based, lobulated 8-mm aneurysm of the ACOM (well visualized on the VRT image presented). This was embolized using microcoils without complication, with images shown from the DSA exam both prior to and immediately following occlusion. Eighteen months later, the patient presented for a follow-up MR. The axial T2-weighted scan is unrevealing, as the signal void could be due to the coiling or represent a flow void. The AP projection from the MIP of the TOF MRA reveals a small area of recanalization (*asterisk*) at the base of the prior aneurysm. Close inspection of TOF images in all aneurysm MR follow-up exams is mandated.

of a vessel, across the neck of an aneurysm. Flow into the aneurysm is disrupted, in theory without interference to flow in the parent vessel or into branch vessels crossed by the stent. Current designs cover about 30% of the surface area. Reduction of flow into the aneurysm leads to thrombosis, which typically takes months, eventually with endothelialization of the stent. This new endothelium is interrupted only by the ostia of branch vessels. In this emergent field, experience is greatest with the Pipeline device, which is approved for clinical use in both the United States and Europe. Placement of a flow diverter may be combined with coiling of the aneurysm. The incidence of adverse events, in published studies to date, is low; however, these include aneurysm rupture and branch artery occlusion.

■ Intracranial Aneurysms by Location

Cavernous ICA Aneurysms

Most cavernous carotid aneurysms are discovered incidentally. The vast majority of patients are women. Symptoms may be related to cranial nerve involvement or a carotid-cavernous fistula. Large aneurysms within the cavernous sinus can cause symptoms due to compression of the cranial nerves that run therein (**Fig. 5.9**). The most common symptoms are diplopia, due to involvement of the oculomotor nerves, and pain, due to involvement of the trigeminal nerve. In a published series, pain and diplopia were noted to resolve spontaneously without treatment in about half of all patients.

Rupture is seen in well less than 10%. Rupture often produces a carotid-cavernous fistula. Subarachnoid hemorrhage is rare. With rupture and an associated carotid-cavernous fistula, possible symptoms include a pulsatile bruit, exophthalmos, ophthalmoplegia, and diminished vision.

Paraclinoid ICA Aneurysms

These arise between the distal dural ring and the origin of PCOM. There are three major types: aneurysms that arise from the ophthalmic or superior hypophyseal artery origins and carotid cave aneurysms. Carotid cave aneurysms arise from the clinoid segment of the ICA (proximal to the origin of the ophthalmic artery) and project medially (**Fig. 5.10**, Parts 1 and 2). These are not infrequently noted incidentally on TOF MRA of the circle of Willis. It is difficult to determine on the basis of imaging whether such an aneurysm is intra- or extradural.

Ophthalmic artery aneurysms typically project superiorly and medially. Of symptomatic lesions, half present with visual

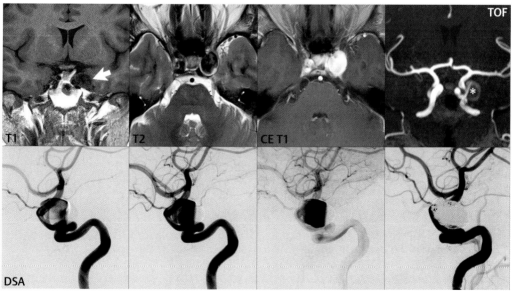

Fig. 5.9 Cavernous carotid aneurysm. On a coronal fast spin echo T1-weighted image, the aneurysm is seen as a flow void (*arrow*), with local mass effect. The appearance is similar on the T2-weighted axial image. Postcontrast, using a short TE GRE T1-weighted scan, there is opacification (enhancement, demonstration of filling) of the aneurysm. The neck of the aneurysm is small, reflected in part by the jet (flow, *asterisk*) seen on the coronal thick MIP TOF MRA, with the majority of the aneurysm low SI due to delayed filling. The aneurysm measured 25 mm, which by definition is the cutoff for a giant aneurysm. The lateral projection from DSA, with three time-sequential images illustrated from a single contrast injection, confirms the jet and delayed filling (with contrast noted layering anteriorly within the aneurysm, following washout from the intracranial vasculature). The aneurysm was occluded using platinum microcoils, with the final DSA image obtained following embolization.

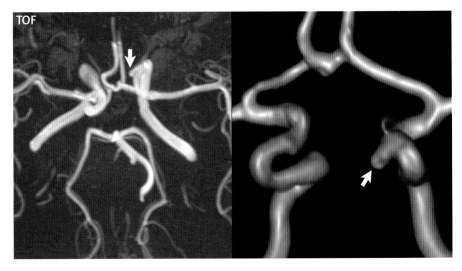

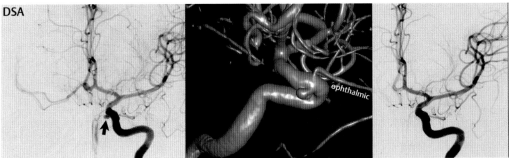

Fig. 5.10 Carotid cave aneurysm. A small, broad-based, 4-mm-diameter aneurysm (*white and black arrows*) is seen well on both TOF MRA (Part 1) and DSA (Part 2), occurring just distal to the anterior genu of the left internal carotid artery (ICA) and projecting medially. In this region, the ICA has exited the cavernous sinus, having passed through the proximal dural ring, but is not yet intradural (subarachnoid) in location, having not passed through the distal dural ring. The origin of the ophthalmic artery, which in 90% of patients is intradural, is seen well on both modalities, distal to the aneurysm. Complete occlusion was achieved using platinum microcoils, as illustrated on the final DSA image.

symptoms (due to impingement on the optic nerve) and half with subarachnoid hemorrhage. Coiling is preferred due to the risk of visual loss with surgery (**Fig. 5.11**). However, relatively high recurrence rates are reported after coiling.

Superior hypophyseal artery aneurysms arise from inferomedial aspect of the ICA, projecting also in this direction. This vessel arises just distal to the ophthalmic artery. Surgical access is technically challenging.

Supraclinoid ICA Aneurysms

PCOM aneurysms typically project inferiorly and laterally (**Fig. 5.12**, Parts 1 and 2).

Both surgery and endovascular treatment are relatively straightforward. A small percentage (< 10%) of all unruptured intracranial aneurysms present with mass effect, typically cranial nerve palsy. Of these, oculomotor palsy due to impingement on the third cranial nerve by a PCOM aneurysm is the most common. Rupture of a PCOM aneurysm is a common cause of subarachnoid hemorrhage. In this instance, the epicenter of acute subarachnoid blood is typically located laterally in the suprasellar and ambient cisterns.

Anterior choroidal artery aneurysms tend to be small, projecting inferiorly and posteriorly. Preservation of the artery (during treatment of the aneurysm) is critical, since the vessel

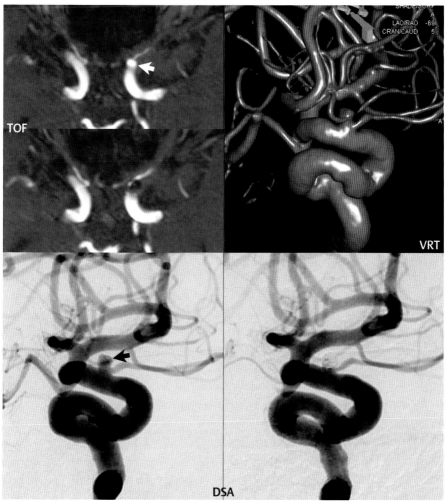

Fig. 5.11 Small ophthalmic artery aneurysm, endovascular therapy. Thin axial MIPs from two TOF MRA exams are presented, prior to (upper) and following (lower) coiling. A small aneurysm (*white arrow*) involving the origin of the left ophthalmic artery is noted prior to treatment. On the subsequent MRA, a signal void is noted in the region of the prior aneurysm, slightly larger in size than the actual area coiled (due to magnetic susceptibility effects). Note the preservation of flow in the left ophthalmic artery. The VRT image from DSA demonstrates the incorporation of the origin of the left ophthalmic artery by this small, 3-mm, sessile aneurysm. Using a temporary remodeling mesh (due to the wide neck), two platinum microcoils were placed, with complete thrombosis of the aneurysm. Lateral DSA projections demonstrate well the aneurysm (*black arrow*) prior to and following microcoil placement.

supplies the internal capsule (**Fig. 5.13**). At the carotid terminus, the internal carotid artery branches into the MCA and ACA. Aneurysms here are not uncommon and tend to be large.

Anterior Cerebral Artery Aneurysms

As with all intracranial aneurysms, screening MR is very effective for diagnosis/visualization of nonruptured anterior communicating artery (ACOM) aneurysms (**Fig. 5.14**). Attention to the characteristic areas where aneurysms occur intracranially is mandatory in exam interpretation.

Rupture of an ACOM aneurysm, like that of a PCOM aneurysm, is a common cause of subarachnoid hemorrhage. Also in common with PCOM aneurysms, both surgery and endovascular treatment are relatively uncomplicated.

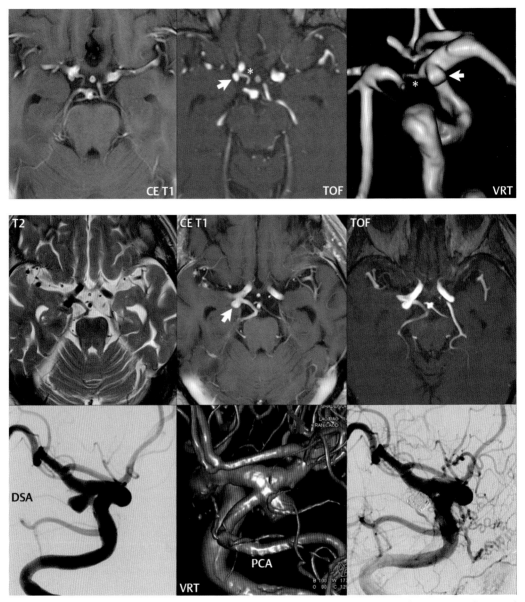

Fig. 5.12 Unruptured PCOM aneurysms, two examples. (Part 1) This 4-mm aneurysm arises at the origin of PCOM, but without incorporation thereof. The aneurysm can be identified on the 4-mm post-contrast axial T1-weighted screening exam. It is better visualized on the thin MIP TOF MRA (*arrow*), with the origin of the right PCOM (*asterisk*) clearly separate. The aneurysm is broad based and well depicted by VRT, with that image being derived from the TOF MRA. (Part 2) A slightly larger 5-mm broad-based PCOM aneurysm is depicted, seen as a flow void on the axial T2-weighted scan, due to contrast enhancement on the short TE GRE axial T1-weighted exam, and with high SI due to flow on the axial thin MIP TOF MRA. Note that this aneurysm completely incorporates the vessel (a fetal origin PCA) in this instance. Lateral views are presented from DSA, both prior to and following coiling (with complete occlusion of the aneurysm), together with VRT derived from the DSA.

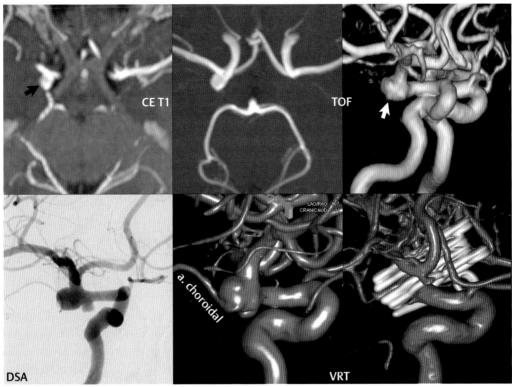

Fig. 5.13 Anterior choroidal artery aneurysm, treated by surgical clipping. A broad-based 8-mm aneurysm (*black arrow*) is identified on the right in the region of the carotid terminus on an axial thin section image (MP-RAGE). Improved depiction of the aneurysm (*white arrow*) is provided by VRT of the TOF MRA. DSA identifies two aneurysms, both along the inferior wall of the distal segment of the supraclinoid internal carotid artery. The anterior choroidal artery is noted to arise from the distal tip of the aneurysm, which is best seen on the VRT image, making endovascular treatment options unacceptable. DSA following surgery shows complete occlusion of the aneurysm by four fenestrated clips (with a fifth clip occluding the smaller aneurysm) and reconstruction of the anterior choroidal artery.

With acute rupture, hemorrhage occurring in the pericallosal cistern is somewhat specific, with hemorrhage inferomedially in the frontal lobe less so.

Anterior cerebral artery aneurysms arising distal to the anterior communicating artery are much less common, but still compose a significant percentage (perhaps 5%) of all intracranial aneurysms (**Fig. 5.15**). Most are small and occur at the A2-A3 junction, being referred to as pericallosal artery aneurysms. Although an azygos ACA (azygous A2 segment) is uncommon, this anatomic variant is strongly associated with aneurysms, specifically at the termination of the A2 segment.

Middle Cerebral Artery Aneurysms

Middle cerebral artery aneurysms (**Fig. 5.16**) are the third most common cause of aneurysmal subarachnoid hemorrhage, in incidence behind ACOM and PCOM artery aneurysms. Acute subarachnoid hemorrhage in the sylvian fissure can occur with internal carotid, PCOM, or MCA aneurysms. Eighty-five percent of MCA aneurysms occur at the bifurcation/trifurcation. More distal aneurysms are likely to be infectious or inflammatory in origin.

Posterior Circulation Aneurysms

Half of all posterior circulation aneurysms are located at the basilar tip. Surgery is difficult

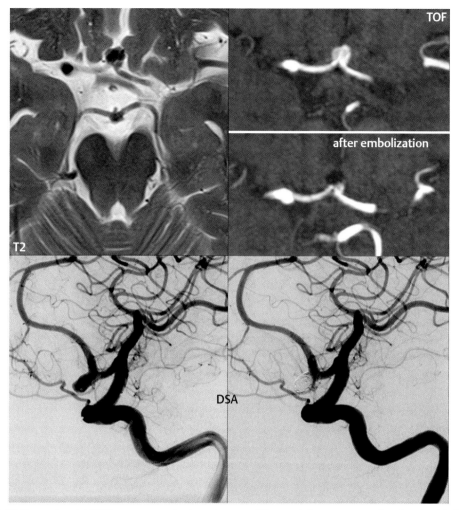

Fig. 5.14 Nonruptured ACOM aneurysm, prior to and following coiling. On an axial 4-mm T2-weighted scan at 3 T, a round flow void is seen in the expected location of the ACOM. An axial thin MIP from the TOF MRA confirms the presence of an aneurysm, with the postcoiling TOF exam (obtained 2 days later) demonstrating nonfilling and the presence of a signal void due to the platinum coils. On DSA, the aneurysm measured 6 mm in greatest dimension and was located at the junction of the ACOM with the A2 segment. Comparison of images from the DSA, prior to and immediately following coiling, reveals complete occlusion.

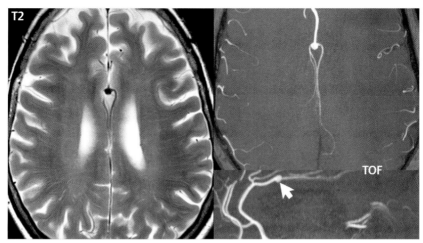

Fig. 5.15 Pericallosal aneurysm. A 5-mm aneurysm is noted involving the A3 segment of a single (unpaired) pericallosal artery, with incorporation of the A4 branches. The aneurysm is well visualized, as a flow void, on a single axial 4-mm T2-weighted scan centered on the lesion. TOF MRA, with thin axial and sagittal MIPs shown, depicts well the aneurysm (*arrow*) at the juncture of the (single) A3 and (paired) A4 segments.

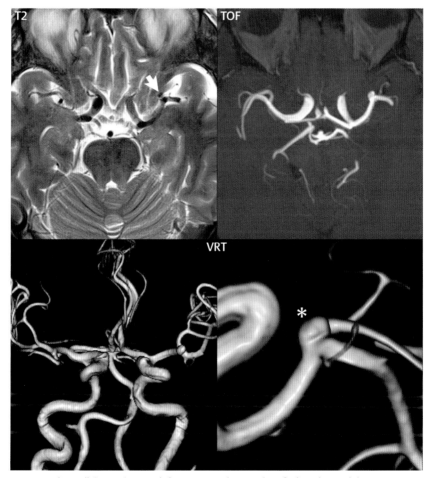

Fig. 5.16 Unruptured, small (4 mm), MCA bifurcation aneurysm. Close inspection of the MCA bifurcation on a screening axial T2-weighted scan at 3 T reveals a small aneurysm projecting anteriorly (*white arrow*). This is better identified on the axial thin MIP TOF MRA. Volume rendering technique (VRT), applied to the TOF MRA exam, depicts well this broad-based aneurysm (*asterisk*), which arises from the MCA bifurcation on the left.

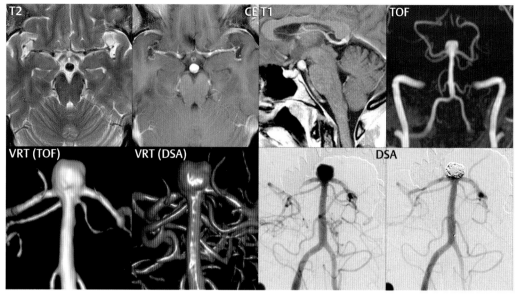

Fig. 5.17 Basilar tip aneurysm. On the axial T2-weighted scan, a flow void is noted in the expected location of, but larger in diameter than, the normal basilar tip. On axial and sagittal contrast-enhanced T1-weighted scans, there is uniform enhancement of this structure, which on the sagittal exam is noted to be located at the terminus of the basilar artery. The exam was obtained at 3 T, with the postcontrast enhancement of arterial structures due to the use of a short TE 2D gradient echo technique. A thick MIP coronal projection from the TOF MRA exam demonstrates well this asymptomatic basilar tip aneurysm. The VRT from the MR exam reveals incorporation of the origins of the posterior cerebral arteries bilaterally. The dimensions of this aneurysm were $8 \times 7 \times 8$ mm^3, with a broad base—the width of the neck being 5 mm. The VRT from the DSA exam once again depicts the aneurysm in 3D, with a similar appearance to the MR. Frontal DSA projections of the posterior circulation using a vertebral injection demonstrate the aneurysm both prior to and following occlusion with platinum microcoils.

in this location, with endovascular treatment (coiling) the technique of choice (**Fig. 5.17**). The most characteristic distribution of blood is that of perimesencephalic or interpeduncular cisternal hemorrhage in combination with midbrain hemorrhage.

Posterior cerebral artery, superior cerebellar artery, basilar trunk, anterior inferior cerebellar artery, and vertebrobasilar junction aneurysms are all uncommon. Each represents less than 1% of all intracranial aneurysms. Aneurysms at the origin of the posterior inferior cerebellar artery (PICA), from the vertebral artery, account for about 2% of all intracranial aneurysms (**Fig. 5.18**). Due to this incidence, acquisition of time of flight MRA exams in all cases to include the origin of PICA is strongly suggested, with one major purpose of this exam being screening for aneurysms. Distal PICA aneurysms are much less common, occurring at branch points and curves in the vessel. Association with AVMs or dural AV fistulas (AVFs) is common.

■ Subarachnoid Hemorrhage

About 80% of nontraumatic subarachnoid hemorrhage (SAH) occurs due to a ruptured aneurysm. Thus 20% of patients with spontaneous SAH will have a negative angiographic workup. Within this latter category of patients, there are two important entities to remember. The first is perimesencephalic nonaneurysmal subarachnoid hemorrhage. In this entity, subarachnoid hemorrhage is present anterior to the pons, often in an asymmetric pattern and within the ambient cistern as well. The bleed is thought to be venous in origin. Neurologic changes are uncommon and the clinical outcome excellent. The second entity is reversible cerebrovascular constriction syndrome, seen

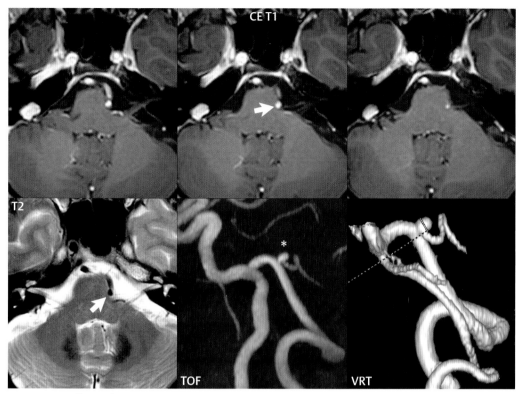

Fig. 5.18 Small saccular PICA origin aneurysm. Aneurysms at the origin of PICA from the vertebral artery are uncommon, comprising 0.5 to 3% of all intracranial aneurysms. Three adjacent, thin section (1 mm), axial, contrast-enhanced, T1-weighted sections demonstrate an aneurysm (*arrow*) arising from the vertebral artery and extending superiorly. The 4-mm, axial, T2-weighted scan depicts the aneurysm as a small flow void (*arrow*). Thick MIP and VRT projections from the TOF MRA exam visualize well this 4-mm aneurysm (*asterisk*), which extends superiorly and incorporates the origin of PICA.

primarily in women. Presentation with a thunderclap headache is common. Up to a third of patients with this syndrome will have SAH. On angiography, whether DSA or MRA, pathognomonic segmental vasoconstriction is seen. Prognosis is very good, with symptoms and angiographic findings resolving within a week. Other important, though much less common, causes of SAH include AVM, dural AVF, disorders of coagulation, cocaine, vasculitis, and venous sinus thrombosis. In addition, it should always be kept in mind that the most common cause of SAH is trauma (**Fig. 5.19**, Parts 1 and 2).

Aneurysmal Subarachnoid Hemorrhage

Depending on the part of the world, the annual incidence of acute SAH from an aneurysm can be as high as 50 per 100,000 population.

The incidence increases with age, and rates are higher in women, African Americans, and Hispanics.

The classic clinical presentation is sudden onset of "the worst headache of my life." Other characteristic symptoms that should raise the suspicion of acute SAH from an aneurysm include nausea and vomiting, diminished consciousness, and focal neurologic findings. The presentation on CT is that of prominent hyperdense blood in the subarachnoid space, commonly also intraventricular. CTA assumes today the primary role in the workup of spontaneous SAH, having replaced catheter angiography (**Fig. 5.20**, Parts 1 and 2). The latter is still indicated in cases of acute SAH not explained by CTA.

In the acute setting, with a small ruptured aneurysm, it is well known that a small percentage of patients can have a normal X-ray

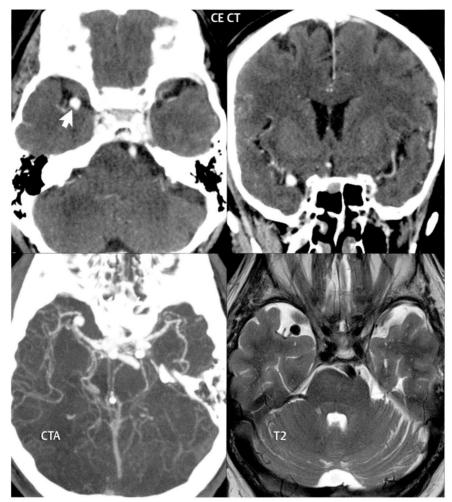

Fig. 5.19 MCA aneurysm, with posttraumatic subarachnoid hemorrhage. (Part 1) A small round enhancing lesion (*white arrow*) is identified on the right along the course of the middle cerebral artery on axial and coronal postcontrast CT images. CTA (thin MIP) confirms the diagnosis of an aneurysm, which measured 6 mm and is located at the MCA bifurcation on the right. As might be anticipated, the aneurysm is also well seen on a precontrast axial T2-weighted scan, as a round flow void. (*continued*)

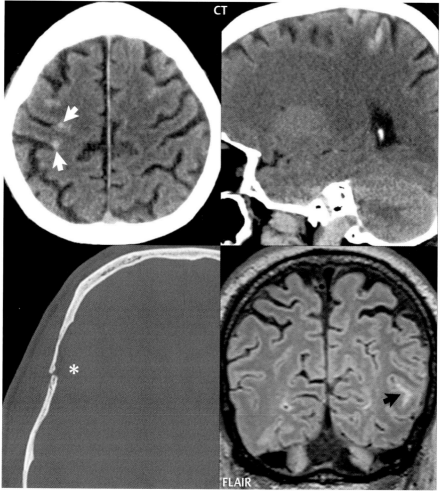

Fig. 5.19 *(Continued)*(Part 2) There are many etiologies to subarachnoid hemorrhage, with rupture of an aneurysm being just one. This patient sustained a head injury due to a fall, the reason for admission and diagnostic imaging. Several small areas of subarachnoid hemorrhage (*white arrows*) were noted, traumatic in etiology, bilaterally, with that illustrated on axial and sagittal unenhanced CT reformats near the vertex. The pattern of hemorrhage is not one typically associated with a ruptured aneurysm and is indeed that commonly seen following trauma. The severity of the injury is revealed in part by the mildly displaced fracture (*asterisk*) of the calvarium on the right, illustrated on an axial CT image reformatted with a bone algorithm (lower left hand corner image). Note the overlying soft tissue prominence. The FLAIR coronal scan also identifies the subarachnoid hemorrhage, here seen as abnormal high signal intensity within a sulcus (*black arrow*) in the left occipital lobe.

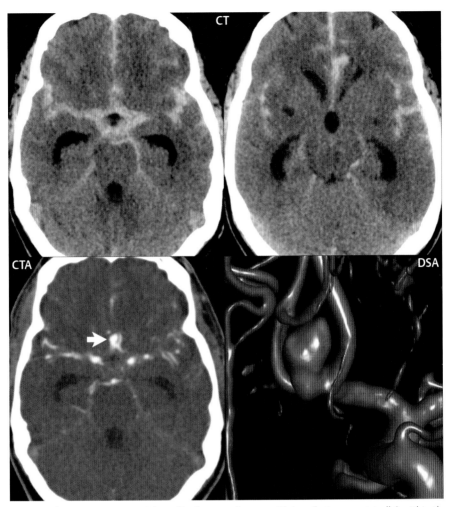

Fig. 5.20 Ruptured ACOM aneurysm, with studies from two patients illustrated. In Part 1, there is extensive acute subarachnoid hemorrhage together with ventricular enlargement, the latter consistent with extraventricular obstructive hydrocephalus (communicating hydrocephalus). Note the prominence of blood along the midline and within the anterior interhemispheric fissure, with less (but symmetrically) within the sylvian fissures, suggestive of an anterior communicating artery (ACOM) aneurysm. A small amount of acute blood is also seen within the inferomedial frontal lobe on the left, also favoring an ACOM aneurysm. CTA identifies the aneurysm (*arrow*), which is well depicted on the subsequent DSA (VRT) study. *(continued)*

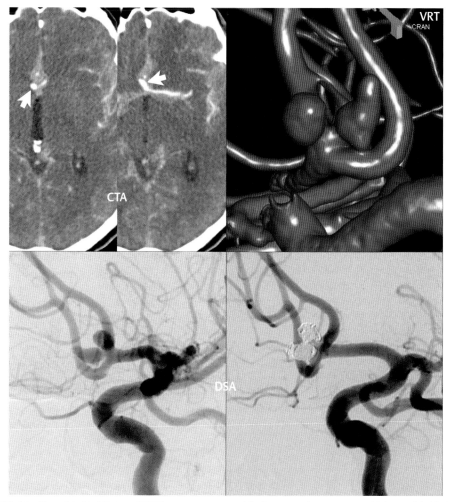

Fig. 5.20 *(Continued)* In Part 2, two ACOM aneurysms (*arrows*) are identified, both on CTA and DSA (VRT). Note the prominent subarachnoid hemorrhage within the anterior interhemispheric fissure, encompassing the aneurysms. The more superior aneurysm is directed medially and superiorly, with the more inferior aneurysm directed medially and anteriorly. Irregularity in shape and an aspect ratio > 1.3 (both present with the second aneurysm, which was felt likely to be the cause of the bleeding) are thought to be predictors of rupture, independent of size and location. The A1 segment of the right anterior cerebral artery is hypoplastic. DSA images from a selective internal carotid artery injection, lateral projection, are also presented prior to and following embolization (with platinum microcoils), with complete occlusion demonstrated.

angiogram. This is presumed to be due to vasospasm, thrombosis, or mass effect, with nonfilling of the aneurysm, despite the abundant subarachnoid blood. It stands to reason that MRA and CTA can also be negative in this instance. Regardless, for angiogram-negative SAH, MR remains a diagnostic option. Repeat angiography (DSA) is indicated if a ruptured aneurysm remains clinically suspect, with the yield of a second such exam as high as 15%.

Up to one-third of patients presenting with a ruptured intracranial aneurysm will die within the first month. Most deaths occur within 2 weeks, and over half occur within 48 hours. Long-term morbidity is substantial. The highest risk of re-bleeding occurs within the first 24 hours (up to 20%). Half of all patients re-bleed within 6 months. Patients with more severe symptoms upon admission and those with larger aneurysms are at greater

risk for re-bleeding. Early treatment of an aneurysm, within 24 hours (prior to the onset of vasospasm), by either surgery or coiling is indicated in order to minimize the risk of re-hemorrhage and possible complications from treatment. After treatment, the risk of recurrent SAH continues to be substantially higher than in the general population.

Hydrocephalus is common following SAH. When evaluating a scan, close inspection of the tips of the temporal horns can be particularly helpful in diagnosing ventricular enlargement (**Fig. 5.21**). Chronic shunt-dependent post-SAH hydrocephalus is also common, occurring in up to half of patients. Seizures, in the acute time period, as well as chronically, are not uncommon (occurring in < 10%).

Symptomatic vasospasm, seen in approximately one fourth of patients, is the major cause of mortality and morbidity

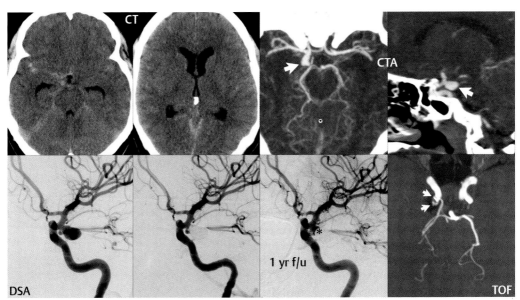

Fig. 5.21 Ruptured PCOM aneurysm, presenting acutely with a moderate headache and neck stiffness (Hess grade 2). On the CT at admission, there is scattered subarachnoid hemorrhage, which was most prominent in the suprasellar cistern on the right. A small amount of blood is noted layering in the atria of the lateral ventricles. Given the patient's age (33 years), there is mild ventricular enlargement, consistent with extraventricular obstructive hydrocephalus, which is easiest to assess by inspection of the size of the tips of the temporal horns. Note the relative absence of blood within the sylvian fissures at the level of the frontal horns of the lateral ventricles. CTA (axial and sagittal thin MIP images) identifies an ovoid aneurysm (*arrow*) at the origin of the PCOM, measuring 15 mm in greatest diameter. The aneurysm is well identified on a lateral view from DSA performed the next day, with images presented both prior to and following coiling using platinum microcoils. On follow-up DSA 1 year later, there is a small area of recanalization (*asterisk*) at the neck of the aneurysm. This can also be visualized on an axial thin MIP from the TOF MRA exam (*small white arrows*), seen within the area of signal void due to the platinum coils.

following SAH. Angiographically, it is defined as a greater than 50% reduction in arterial caliber and involves both large and small intracranial arteries. Vasospasm rarely occurs prior to day 3, is maximal at 1 week, and resolves in most patients by 2 weeks. The presence of red blood cells (RBCs) is necessary for vasospasm to occur, and the timing of the onset of vasospasm correlates with that of RBC lysis. Clinical features include confusion and a decline in consciousness. The more blood present on the CT at presentation, the greater are the likelihood and severity of vasospasm. Catheter angiography remains the gold standard for diagnosis. CTA is excellent for detection of significant vasospasm involving large intracranial vessels. Regional areas of decreased CBF indicative of symptomatic vasospasm can be detected by CT perfusion studies.

The International Subarachnoid Aneurysm Trial (ISAT) was a large, randomized, prospective, multicenter trial evaluating endovascular coiling versus surgical clipping in patients with ruptured intracranial aneurysms. The study began in 1994, with enrollment discontinued in 2002 when interim analysis showed a significant advantage for endovascular coiling. There was a significant reduction in mortality and morbidity in the endovascular group, which also had better cognitive outcomes. However, the re-bleeding rate was greater with coiling. These results apply only to aneurysms that can be treated by either surgery or coiling.

■ Other Aneurysm Subtypes

Infectious Aneurysms

The term *mycotic aneurysm* is used colloquially for all infectious aneurysms, although strictly the term *mycotic* refers to fungal (**Fig. 5.22**). Infectious aneurysms are uncommon, accounting for less than 1% of all intracranial aneurysms. Most mycotic aneurysms are caused by septic emboli. The majority of patients have endocarditis. Other predisposing conditions include meningitis, sinus infection, and cavernous sinus thrombophlebitis. Most present with rupture, and the majority are within the MCA territory. Multiple lesions occur in 20%.

Streptococcus and *Staphylococcus* are the most common causes, with intracranial fungal aneurysms actually rare. Infectious aneurysms and their adjacent vessels are fragile. First-line therapy for unruptured infectious aneurysms is antibiotics. Surgery is reserved for hemorrhagic lesions or lesions that enlarge despite antibiotic therapy (**Fig. 5.23**). Historically, the mortality rate was high, up to 40%, although recent reports describe good outcomes in 80%.

Mycotic aneurysms are usually peripheral in location, in distinction to saccular aneurysms. Serial evaluation (by MR, CTA, or DSA) is recommended to assess for possible enlargement. Conventional CT and MR imaging is nonspecific in regard to appearance, demonstrating a small enhancing lesion with surrounding cerebral edema.

Giant Aneurysms

By definition, a giant aneurysm is one that is ≥ 25 mm in diameter. They can be saccular or fusiform in shape and are more common in the posterior circulation (with other frequent locations including the cavernous and supraclinoid internal carotid artery). They comprise 5% of all intracranial aneurysms and occur in older patients. Intraluminal thrombus is common. The annual rate of rupture is high. Clinical presentation may be due to mass effect (cranial nerve palsies) or rupture (subarachnoid hemorrhage).

In regard to MR technique, there are a few caveats. Giant aneurysms may not be depicted in their entirety on 3D TOF MRA due to slow flow within the aneurysm, and in this instance, correlation with 2D TOF and conventional (non-flow-related) images, or additional contrast-enhanced 3D MRA, can be helpful in delineating the true luminal extent (**Fig. 5.9**). Large aneurysms may also be associated with pulsation artifacts on MR, which can help to confirm the vascular nature of the lesion on conventional T1- and T2-weighted cross-sectional images. On a flow study such as CTA or MRA, the size of even a small saccular aneurysm can be underestimated, due to the presence of thrombus. Comparison of conventional MR scans with source images

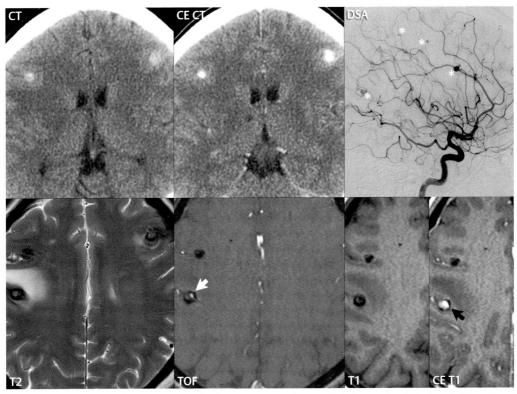

Fig. 5.22 Multiple embolic (mycotic) cerebral aneurysms from a left atrial myxoma. On CT, two small hyperdense foci are noted peripherally in the frontal lobes, with enhancement postcontrast. A lateral projection from an internal carotid artery injection reveals multiple small aneurysms (*asterisks*), predominantly involving distal arterial branches. Some of the lesions are fusiform (tubular) in shape, a characteristic of myxomatous aneurysms, which may also be saccular. Multiple hemorrhagic lesions (with a rim of low SI hemosiderin) are identified on MR, one with substantial associated vasogenic edema. TOF MRA defines a small aneurysm within the latter (*white arrow*). Note that postcontrast, the area of enhancement (*black arrow*) is larger, including both the aneurysm and the inflammation/involvement of the surrounding wall. Associated calcification can also be seen on CT, as in this case.

from the MRA exam improves recognition of thrombus. On rare occasion, with giant aneurysms, layered thrombus is present, which is well visualized on nonangiographic, cross-sectional imaging (**Fig. 5.24**, Parts 1 and 2).

Dolichoectatic and Fusiform Aneurysms

These are uncommon, accounting for < 2% of all intracranial aneurysms. Compression of adjacent structures (brainstem, cranial nerve) is a common cause of symptoms. Rupture is less frequent than with saccular aneurysms. Intraluminal thrombus can be present. Vertebrobasilar dolichoectasia is generally included within this category.

Traumatic Aneurysms

These represent less than 1% of all intracranial aneurysms. Traumatic aneurysms develop 2 to 3 weeks following injury. Typical features include peripheral location, irregular contour, delayed filling, and no apparent neck. Nonpenetrating head injury, specifically due to rapid deceleration, is a more common cause than penetrating injury. Most are found in the anterior circulation. Associated skull fractures are present in 90%. Cortical traumatic aneurysms are seen with calvarial fractures, and petrous or cavernous ICA aneurysms with basilar skull fractures.

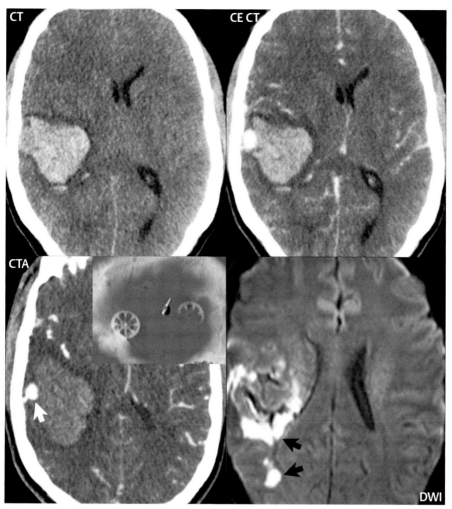

Fig. 5.23 Presentation of an acute parenchymal hematoma in a 39-year-old man. The unenhanced CT reveals a large temporoparietal acute hematoma, with mild circumferential vasogenic edema. There is compression of the right lateral ventricle, in particular the atrium, with right to left midline shift. On the postcontrast scan, a small round enhancing lesion is seen along the lateral border of the hematoma. This is also noted to enhance (*white arrow*) on the CTA, consistent with a mycotic aneurysm. The aneurysm, which proved to be distal M4 in location, was clipped (the *inset* shows a sagittal postoperative image, visualizing the craniotomy and aneurysm clip), and the hematoma evacuated. A postoperative complication is identified on the follow-up MR (DWI), with an acute infarct (abnormal high signal intensity) seen both immediately posterior to the area of evacuation and more distally (*black arrows*). The age of the patient and location of the hematoma are unusual (i.e., not consistent with a hypertensive hemorrhage), and close inspection of the images for clues to the etiology is recommended in such instances.

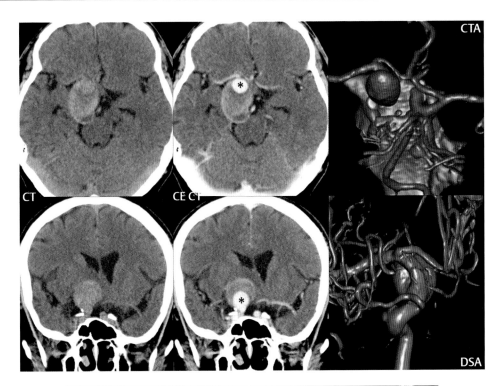

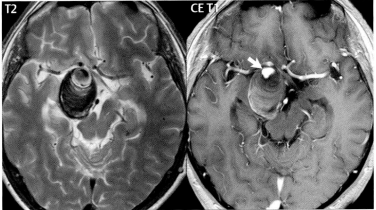

Fig. 5.24 Partially thrombosed giant aneurysm, arising from the posterior wall of the right ICA, distal to the origin of the ophthalmic artery and as the supraclinoid segment begins. Axial and coronal CT reformats are presented (Part 1) prior to and following intravenous contrast administration, depicting the much smaller enhancing, patent portion of the aneurysm (*asterisk*). There is mass effect upon the adjacent brain and vasculature. The patent portion of the aneurysm and the relevant adjacent vessels (note that the aneurysm arises prior to and separate from the carotid terminus) are well depicted on CTA (VRT) and DSA. On MR (Part 2), the clot has a laminated appearance, reflecting the different layers and time frames of thrombosis, which is pathognomonic, but not common, for a partially thrombosed giant aneurysm. The central patent portion (*white arrow*) of the aneurysm is noted to enhance postcontrast.

6 Vascular Malformations and Other Vascular Lesions

◼ Arteriovenous Malformation

An arteriovenous malformation (AVM) consists of a nidus (tangle) of tightly packed dilated, tortuous arteries and veins, without an intervening capillary network, with the result being arteriovenous shunting. It is the most common symptomatic vascular malformation of brain. The risk of hemorrhage is 2 to 4% per year, with each episode having a 30% risk of death. Most lesions present clinically between 20 and 40 years of age and involve peripheral branches of the ACA or MCA. Aneurysms of the feeding arteries (perinidal aneurysms), due to high flow, are seen in less than 10% of cases. AVMs are considered to be congenital in origin; they are one-tenth as common as aneurysms. Hemodynamically, AVMs have high flow and low resistance.

The nidus of an AVM may be compact or somewhat diffuse. They are often pyramidal in shape, with their base along a cortical surface and their apex directed toward a ventricle (**Fig. 6.1**). Although not common, there may

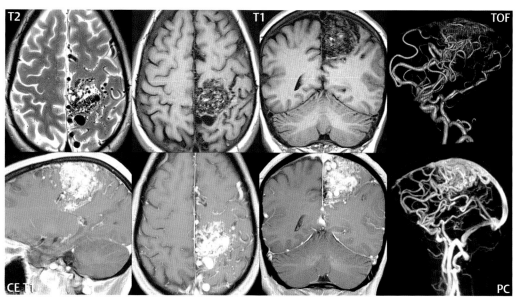

Fig. 6.1 Left paracentral lobule arteriovenous malformation. Flow voids are noted in the left paracentral lobule, together with the precentral, postcentral, and cingulate gyri. There is mild mass effect upon the adjacent brain, best demonstrated on the coronal scans. In regard to MR technique (with the scan performed at 3 T), the precontrast T1-weighted scans are obtained with fast spin echo technique and the postcontrast scans with gradient echo technique. The former allows best visualization of the flow voids, and the latter the best visualization of contrast enhancement in both the feeding arteries and draining veins. TOF MRA will visualize predominately the large feeding arteries, together with partial visualization of the nidus and draining veins. The arterial supply is in this instance primarily from the ACA and MCA, with the venous drainage in part via the superior sagittal sinus. Phase contrast MRA can be used, as illustrated, to achieve improved visualization of the venous drainage. The location of the lesion leaves little to no options regarding possible treatment. The paracentral lobule, a continuation of the pre- and postcentral gyri, is supplied by the ACA and controls both motor and sensory innervation for the contralateral lower extremity.

be hemosiderin staining in the adjacent brain parenchyma due to previous hemorrhage. A total of 65% involve the cerebral hemispheres, 15% the deep midline structures, and 20% the posterior fossa. Most are sporadic in occurrence. Intracranial AVMs occur in about 10% of cases of hereditary hemorrhagic telangiectasia (Rendu-Osler-Weber syndrome).

AVMs are well depicted on conventional, cross-sectional MR imaging (due to flow phenomena), with TOF MRA used to better demonstrate the nidus, enlarged arterial feeding vessels, and enlarged draining veins. On occasion, a small AVM will be visualized only on MR angiography and not well seen on other MR sequences. On precontrast conventional MR scans, multiple serpiginous vessels,

most with low SI due to rapid flow, are typically visualized. Contrast enhancement often provides improved visualization of the nidus, together with the enlarged draining veins (**Fig. 6.2**; **Fig. 6.3**).

Between the large draining veins, there will be preserved normal brain parenchyma. Gliosis is uncommon. There is usually little mass effect, with vasogenic edema unusual. Acute hemorrhage is well visualized on unenhanced CT; however, on such scans, even large AVMs may not be detected. Calcification is seen in the minority of cases. Enhancement on CT (together with CTA) provides visualization of the nidus and large draining veins (**Fig. 6.4**). DSA remains the gold standard for evaluation of an AVM, with one major advantage being

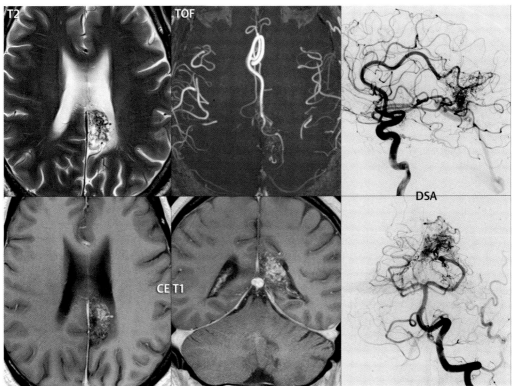

Fig. 6.2 An AVM in the region of the splenium of the corpus callosum on the left, depicted by both MR and DSA. A nidus of small flow voids is noted on the T2-weighted FSE axial scan, with corresponding contrast enhancement on the short TE GRE T1-weighted axial and coronal scans. A thick MIP axial slab from the TOF MRA reveals the arterial supply from the left pericallosal artery (which is increased in diameter). Although not shown, the left PCA was similarly demonstrated by TOF MRA to supply this AVM. DSA confirms, on lateral and frontal views from left internal carotid and vertebral artery injections, the predominant arterial supply from the distal pericallosal artery and branches of the posterior cerebral artery on the left. Although often not obvious on MR (without prior scans), this AVM had been previously partially embolized.

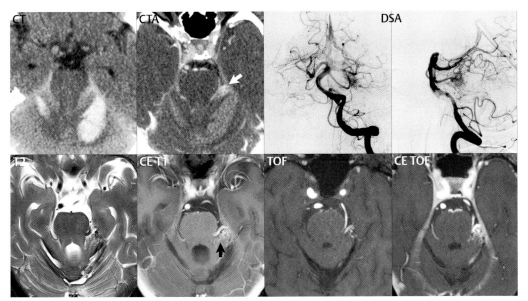

Fig. 6.3 Small left posterior fossa AVM. The patient presented acutely with subarachnoid and intraparenchymal hemorrhage on CT, bilaterally, predominantly confined to the posterior fossa, an unusual pattern for rupture of an intracranial aneurysm. Clinical symptoms included headache, nausea, and dizziness. Although not seen prospectively, close inspection of the CTA reveals an ill-defined enhancing lesion (*white arrow*), perhaps with a tangle of small vessels, in the left ambient cistern. DSA, with frontal and lateral projections illustrated, was performed the following day, revealing a small AVM predominantly supplied by the left superior cerebellar artery. MR performed a week later reveals substantial resorption of the cerebellar hemorrhages, with residual hemosiderin along the rim of each on the T2-weighted image. A small tangle of enhancing vessels is identified postcontrast (*black arrow*), together with a large posterior mesencephalic draining vein (draining subsequently into the basal vein of Rosenthal). Contrast-enhanced TOF MRA, as illustrated, can provide substantially improved depiction of the involved vasculature, in comparison to standard TOF MRA, for AVMs (and, in some instances, also for aneurysms).

the clarification of feeding vessels and draining veins (**Fig. 6.5**). For example, for a convexity lesion, contributions from the ACA and MCA can be distinguished. This can also be done currently by MR, but remains a topic for further research and development.

The risk of hemorrhage from an AVM, from the literature, is 2 to 4% per year. The risk of re-bleeding is increased for several years following a prior hemorrhage. Hemorrhage is the most common presenting symptom (seen in half of all cases) (**Fig. 6.6**; **Fig. 6.7**, Parts 1 and 2), followed by seizures (seen in one-quarter).

Treatment includes surgery, radiosurgery, and embolization. Asymptomatic lesions, difficult to treat lesions, and patients at high risk for complications warrant conservative treatment. Lesions are stratified according to surgical risk by the Spetzler-Martin grading system, which assigns points relative to size,

location, and venous drainage. Lower grade lesions have lower permanent morbidity and mortality following surgery (for example, with permanent morbidity < 5% and mortality < 4% in Spetzler-Martin grades I-III). Surgery can be delayed following hemorrhage, given that AVMs do not have the high, immediate risk of rehemorrhage that aneurysms do. Either intraoperative or postoperative DSA should always be performed to confirm complete obliteration of the lesion. Although uncommon, cerebral edema can occur after surgery and can also be seen with embolization. Surgery may carry a higher cure rate and a lower rehemorrhage risk when compared to radiosurgery.

Radiosurgery delivers a high radiation dose to the isocenter, with a substantially lower dose to nontargeted structures. Current treatment systems include the Gamma Knife and linear accelerator platforms (e.g., the X-Knife

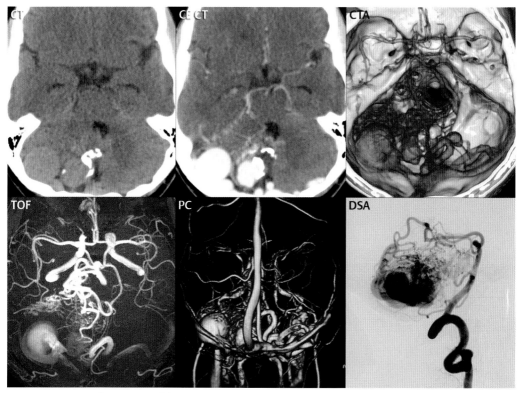

Fig. 6.4 Posterior fossa AVM. Although AVMs can be difficult to detect on unenhanced CT, calcifications, as present with this lesion, are not uncommon and can be a key for diagnosis. There is prominent mass effect upon the adjacent cerebellum, together with mild compression of the fourth ventricle. Both the CTA and the TOF exam demonstrate the arterial inflow to be primarily from the PCA, SCA, AICA, and PICA on the right. The venous outflow is predominately via the right and left transverse sinuses, with a giant venous varix seen on the right.

and the CyberKnife). Radiotherapy causes endothelial damage, leading eventually to stenosis of the vessels in the treated area and subsequent occlusion. This approach is minimally invasive, low risk (but specifically not free of complications, with permanent neurologic deficits seen in 5%), and effective for smaller lesions (≤ 3 cm). Its disadvantage is that obliteration is delayed, occurring over 2 to 3 years following treatment.

Embolization can be performed for palliation (treatment of part of the lesion) or prior to surgery (**Fig. 6.8**, Parts 1 and 2). The latter is performed to reduce the volume of the nidus and to occlude feeders that might be difficult to reach by surgery. Cure rates (complete obliteration) are low for treatment of AVMs with embolization alone (5–10%) (**Fig. 6.9**). This is likely due to the fact that few AVMs have a single pedicle, or just a few pedicles, that can be safely embolized. Embolization materials include polyvinyl alcohol, *N*-butyl-2-cyanoacrylate, and Onyx.

Associated aneurysms are found in less than 10% of AVMs. These may involve feeding arteries (perinidal) (**Fig. 6.5**) or be intranidal, with the latter distinguished from venous varices on DSA by their visualization in the arterial phase. The risk of hemorrhage from an AVM is increased by the presence of an associated aneurysm.

Large (Spetzler-Martin grade IV-V), as well as giant (> 6 cm), AVMs are difficult to treat. Morbidity and mortality with surgery are high. Partial treatment appears not to reduce the risk of hemorrhage; thus, any treatment should be aimed at eventual complete obliteration.

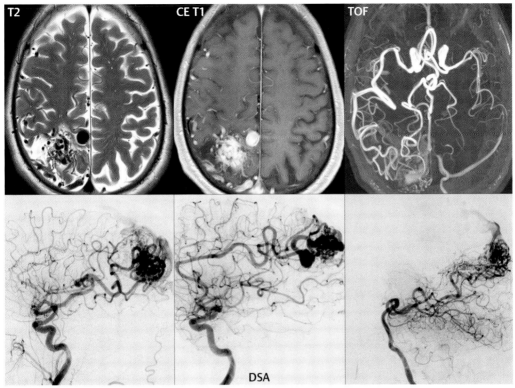

Fig. 6.5 Large right parietal AVM. A tangle of flow voids is noted on the T2-weighted scan, lying within the intraparietal sulcus, with the large nidus best identified on the postcontrast T1-weighted scan. Although focal atrophy is present, note the absence of associated gliosis, despite the size of this AVM. A large round flow void is identified medially, shown by subsequent imaging (and DSA) to be an aneurysm along a feeding vessel. These are seen in less than 10% of AVMs, are commonly multiple, and are at risk for rupture. The TOF MRA reveals an enlarged right MCA, left ACA, and right PCA, all feeding this AVM. The vascular supply is confirmed by lateral DSA projections obtained from right and left ICA injections, along with an injection of the posterior circulation. The large aneurysm is identified on DSA to involve the distal left ACA.

Cerebral proliferative angiopathy (diffuse cerebral angiomatosis) is a rare vascular malformation with several distinguishing characteristics from a classic AVM. These include large size (lobar or hemispheric), absence of dominant feeders and large (and/or early) draining veins, additional meningeal artery involvement, and normal brain intermingled between vessels.

▓ Dural Arteriovenous Fistula

A dural arteriovenous fistula (dAVF) is an acquired vascular malformation of the brain that is most commonly seen involving the transverse and/or sigmoid sinus (and most often on the left). The etiology is believed to be occlusion of a venous sinus, with recanalization along the walls of the sinus leading to numerous direct connections between small feeding arteries and venous drainage (**Fig. 6.10**). Clinical complications include venous infarction, parenchymal hemorrhage (classically with lesions that cause retrograde leptomeningeal cortical venous flow), and subdural hematoma. On MR and enhanced CT, enlarged, superficial, dural-based veins are seen, without a parenchymal nidus.

Symptoms and physical findings with a dAVF are variable, with pulsatile tinnitus most common. dAVFs are the most frequent cause of pulsatile tinnitus, followed by

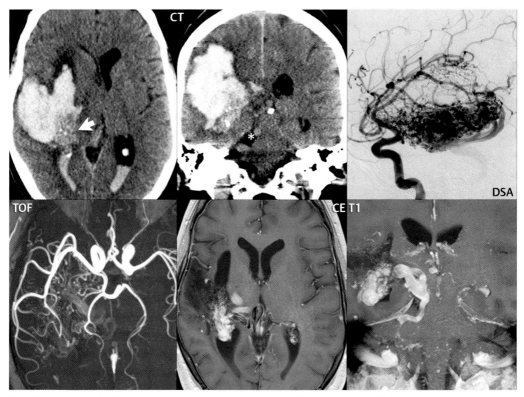

Fig. 6.6 Large retrolenticular AVM, presenting acutely with hemorrhage, but evident due to its size on unenhanced CT performed in the emergency department. On presentation (CT), a large, acute, parenchymal hematoma is noted on the right, traversing the temporal and parietal lobes. There is prominent mass effect, some associated vasogenic edema, and abundant intraventricular blood. Medial, posterior, and inferior to the hemorrhage is an area of intermediate density (*white arrow*), with punctate calcifications, suggestive of a large AVM. In the perimesencephalic cistern on the right, a large serpiginous draining vein (*asterisk*) is noted, consistent with this diagnosis. DSA performed in the acute setting reveals a large AVM, which was supplied by the anterior and posterior choroidal as well as the lenticulostriate arteries. Venous drainage was in part by a dilated basal vein of Rosenthal as well as a tortuous, dilated perimesencephalic vein on the right, the latter draining into the superior petrosal sinus. The latter corresponds to the large vein identified on CT. The bottom row of images, from MR, was acquired 1 year later. A thick MIP axial slab from the TOF MRA again demonstrates feeders from both the anterior and posterior circulation on the right. The nidus and a part of the venous drainage are seen on the postcontrast axial T1-weighted scan (performed with a short TE GRE T1-weighted technique at 3 T, which maximizes visualization of both large and small arteries and veins). Note also the extensive cystic encephalomalacia (with low SI), residual from the prior hemorrhage. A thin MIP of the 2D coronal contrast-enhanced T1-weighted scan depicts part of the nidus and more effectively displays a portion of the venous drainage medially.

atherosclerotic carotid stenosis and carotid cavernous fistulas. A bruit can be heard in up to half of patients. Hydrocephalus may be present due to venous hypertension interfering with CSF absorption. Like AVMs and cavernous malformations, a dAVF can be a cause of intracranial hemorrhage (**Fig. 6.11**). This is more common with leptomeningeal venous drainage, stenosis or occlusion of the associated venous sinuses, and variceal or aneurysmal venous dilatation. White matter changes (T2 hyperintensity) may be observed on MR due to venous hypertension, with restricted diffusion in brain affected by retrograde cortical venous flow.

Digital subtraction angiography is the definitive technique for diagnosis. The most important goal of angiography is to determine if

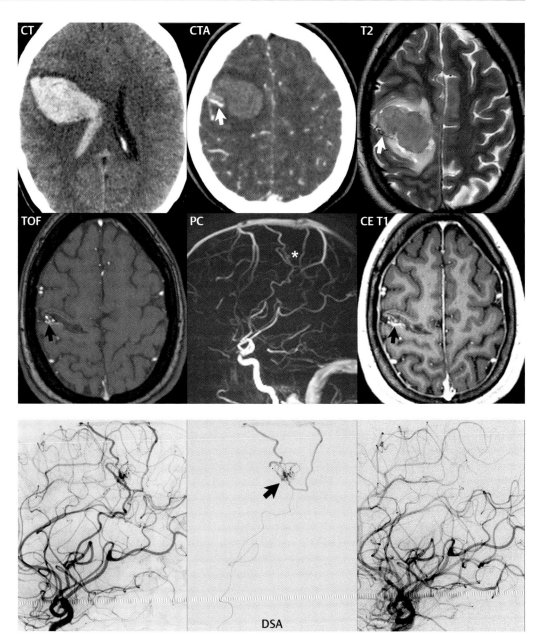

Fig. 6.7 Acute parenchymal hemorrhage, with a small underlying AVM noted on follow-up MR obtained 6 months following presentation (with the interval time allowing for resolution of mass effect and near complete resorption of the hematoma). At presentation on CT, and 6 days later on MR, a large frontoparietal parenchymal hematoma (with extravasation into the lateral ventricle) is noted with mild surrounding vasogenic edema (Part 1). Although not noted prospectively, in retrospect on the CTA, there is the question of an abnormal vein (*white arrow*) immediately posterior and lateral to the hematoma and, on the MR, both a small tangle of flow voids and the associated slightly prominent vein (*white arrow*). A common recommendation is to re-evaluate the patient on MR after a sufficient time interval to allow resorption of the hematoma, which was done in this instance. On that follow-up exam, a small tangle of vessels is noted immediately adjacent and lateral to the small residual fluid cleft on the TOF MRA (*black arrow*) and on phase contrast MRA (*asterisk*), which is noted to enhance postcontrast (*black arrow*), with the latter exam also demonstrating again the slightly enlarged draining vein. DSA (Part 2) was subsequently performed, demonstrating this small plexiform AVM in the precentral sulcus, supplied by a branch of the right MCA. The AVM itself (*black arrow*) and its drainage into the superior sagittal sinus via two cortical veins are best demonstrated on the superselective injection. Following embolization of the nidus with polyvinyl alcohol, repeat angiography shows complete obliteration of the AVM.

127

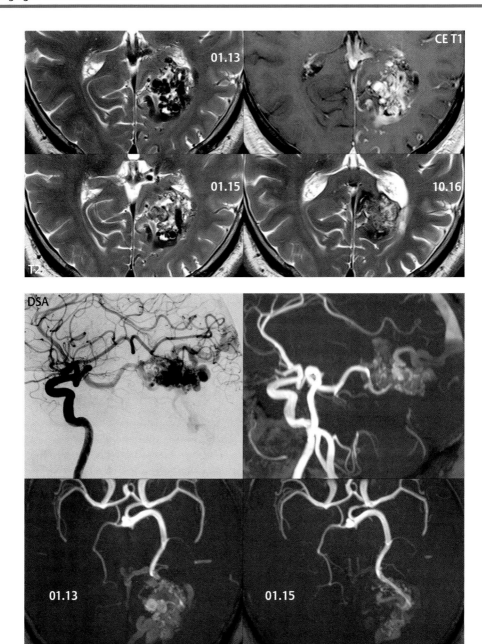

Fig. 6.8 Embolization of an occipital arteriovenous malformation. On the 01.13 MR exam (Part 1), prior to treatment, a tangle of flow voids representing both the nidus and enlarged draining veins is noted medially in the left occipital region, with enhancement postcontrast of the majority of the lesion. On 01.14, several pial branches of the posterior cerebral artery were embolized with cyanoacrylate. On the 01.15 follow-up MR, there is a reduction in flow voids, along with a reduction in caliber of the draining veins above the nidus (not shown). One year and 9 months later, on the 10.16 MR, there is further thrombosis with near complete obliteration of the AVM (note the absence of flow voids). Prior to treatment, a lateral projection from the DSA and a sagittal MIP from the TOF exam (Part 2) depict well this large occipital AVM, with supply by the PCA (as well as from the anterior circulation via a large PCOM) and drainage into the superior sagittal sinus. Note the reduction in the nidus and as well as the large draining veins in comparing the axial thick MIPs from the TOF MRAs prior to (01.13) and following (01.15) the partial embolization.

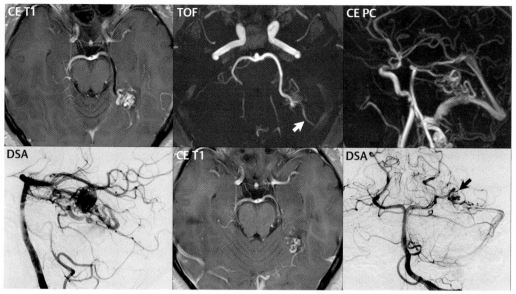

Fig. 6.9 Left posterior parahippocampal AVM. On the postcontrast axial T1-weighted scan, the nidus of this AVM is well visualized, together with its primary arterial supply from the left posterior cerebral artery (seen as a flow void due to fast flow). A small amount of hemosiderin is present, with low signal intensity on this 2D gradient echo scan, adjacent to the nidus, consistent with prior hemorrhage. The thick MIP TOF axial section illustrates both the arterial supply as well as the drainage via a superficial cortical vein (*white arrow*) into the left transverse sinus. The contrast-enhanced PC thick MIP sagittal projection depicts well both the nidus and the enlarged draining veins, as seen in comparison to the lateral DSA projection. Following embolization, there was complete obliteration of the lesion (image not shown). On the follow-up axial postcontrast MR obtained at 1 year, a small nidus of enhancement is visualized, consistent with partial recanalization. This recurrence (*black arrow*) is confirmed on the frontal projection from the subsequent DSA, with the lesion then embolized for a second time.

retrograde leptomeningeal venous drainage is present. Tortuous, engorged veins seen only in the venous phase are indicative of venous congestion and favor retrograde leptomeningeal venous drainage. DSA also allows assessment of the arterial feeders and whether venous outflow obstruction (stenosis or thrombosis) is present. Prominent pial vessels on MR suggest the diagnosis, although a normal MR does not exclude a dAVF. CTA may also show some dAVFs. Borden type I dAVFs (which drain directly into a meningeal vein or dural venous sinus) are considered benign (**Fig. 6.12**).

Types II and III (which either have retrograde drainage into subarachnoid veins or drain directly so) are considered aggressive, with significant risk of hemorrhage or non-hemorrhagic neurologic deficits (due to intracranial venous hypertension). In general, the most effective treatment of a dAVF is by endovascular means. Transvenous techniques,

with obliteration of the draining vein, carry the highest success rate for long-term obliteration, with preservation of normal venous drainage critical. Embolization is performed primarily for dAVFs with aggressive characteristics, although it can be used to alleviate symptoms such as pulsatile tinnitus in benign lesions. Conservative management is reasonable in Borden type I lesions. Intermittent manual compression (of the pulsatile occipital artery) has been shown to cause occlusion in one-quarter of cases within 4 to 6 weeks.

◼ Carotid-Cavernous Fistula

There are two types of carotid-cavernous fistulas (CCFs), "direct" and "indirect." Most direct CCFs are traumatic in etiology, secondary to skull base fracture. A less common cause (20%) is rupture of an aneurysm of the

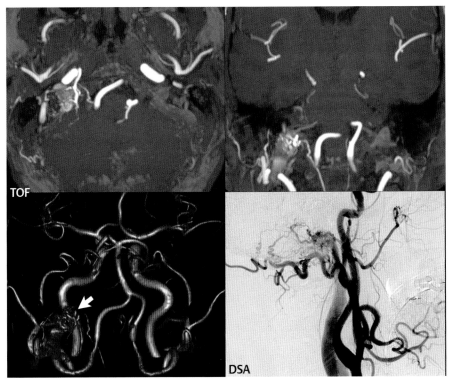

Fig. 6.10 Dural arteriovenous fistula. Thick MIP axial and coronal reformats from a TOF MRA, together with the volume-rendered 3D PA projection depict a complex dural arteriovenous fistula (*arrow*) at the junction of the sigmoid sinus and the jugular bulb in this patient with tinnitus. The fistula was supplied primarily by the ascending pharyngeal artery (from the external carotid artery). The lesion is well seen on a lateral DSA projection from a common carotid artery injection and was subsequently embolized.

internal carotid artery within the cavernous sinus. Direct CCFs are high-flow lesions. Indirect CCFs are low-flow, nontraumatic acquired lesions, representing an AVF of the cavernous sinus with branches either of the external carotid artery or the cavernous carotid artery. With direct CCFs, findings include proptosis (with pulsating exophthalmos clinically), dilatation of the superior ophthalmic vein(s), and enlargement of the cavernous sinus(es) (**Fig. 6.13**, Parts 1 and 2). Prominent flow voids will be present in the cavernous sinus on MR. DSA is the definitive exam for diagnosis. On DSA, early filling of the cavernous sinus, together with retrograde filling of the superior ophthalmic vein, can be seen. There may be reduced flow in the internal carotid artery beyond the fistula.

Detection of an indirect CCF on MR and CT can be difficult. Enlargement of the superior ophthalmic vein(s) is perhaps the most consistent and earliest finding. As with other AVFs, postcontrast imaging may demonstrate increased vascularity surrounding one or both cavernous sinuses. Unlike direct CCFs, the cavernous sinuses are typically not as prominent with an indirect CCF. Indirect CCFs are rarely detected by non-DSA imaging before symptoms are observed clinically.

■ Cerebral Cavernous Malformation

A cerebral cavernous malformation (CCM; previously known as a cavernous angioma or hemangioma) histologically consists of a honeycomb of vascular spaces, separated by fibrous strands, without intervening normal brain parenchyma. The prevalence in the general population is 0.5%. A total of 75% of CCMs are supratentorial, with multiplicity common (25%). The latter are

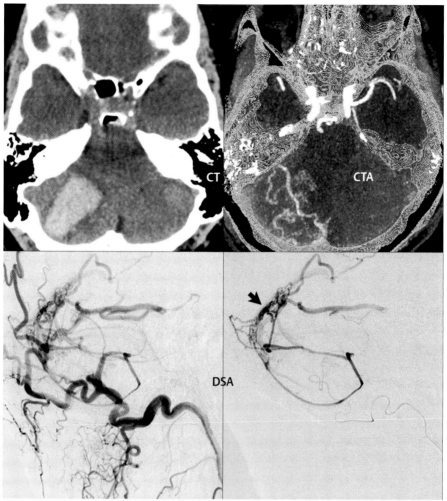

Fig. 6.11 Rupture of a dural arteriovenous (AV) fistula presenting with acute hemorrhage. An unenhanced axial CT depicts a large right cerebellar hematoma, with a thin rim of vasogenic edema. Prominent veins lying just underneath the right tentorium were noted on contrast-enhanced scans. These are well seen on a thin axial MIP from the dual-energy CTA with bone removal. DSA was performed emergently, with two lateral views presented. A dural arteriovenous fistula is visualized (*arrow*), arising near the torcula and supplied by branches of both the occipital and meningeal arteries. The second lateral view is from the super-selective micro-catheterization of the arterial supply from the occipital artery. This dural AV fistula was obliterated by embolization of both arterial feeding vessels using cyanoacrylate.

classified as familial. CCMs are prone to spontaneous hemorrhage. Seizures are the most common presenting symptom. Surgical resection is an option in patients with medically refractory seizures or symptomatic hemorrhagic lesions, if the lesion lies in a surgically accessible location.

As with almost all brain disease (in particular, parenchymal lesions), MR is the modality of choice for detection, differential diagnosis, and evaluation. CCMs are well-circumscribed, lobulated lesions, typically with extensive hemosiderin deposits indicative of previous hemorrhage. On MR, a CCM will have mixed low and high SI on both T1- and T2-weighted images (a "popcorn ball" appearance), with the presence of a complete hemosiderin rim considered important for differential diagnosis. The latter is best visualized on gradient echo T2-weighted images (GRE), as low signal intensity. Susceptibility weighted imaging (SWI) provides a further improvement in visualization of the hemosiderin rim, as

131

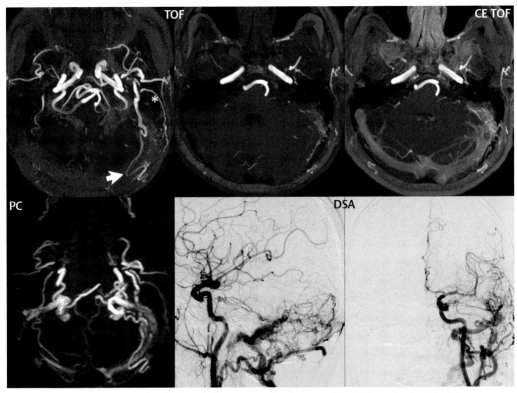

Fig. 6.12 Dural arteriovenous fistula (dAVF), illustrating contrast-enhanced TOF and phase contrast (PC) MRA. The patient presented clinically with tinnitus (synchronous with his pulse). The lesion is located on the left along the wall of the transverse and sigmoid sinuses. Arterial feeders, as demonstrated by a thick axial MIP from the TOF MRA, include the occipital artery (*arrow*) and the posterior auricular artery (*asterisk*), both being branches of the external carotid artery. The fistula itself is best visualized on the thin MIP TOF MRA (middle image, upper row), as a small tangle of vessels in the vicinity of the left transverse sinus. Its specific location is better identified on the CE TOF MRA, due to visualization on that exam of the dural sinuses. Partial thrombosis of the left transverse sinus is also present but poorly demonstrated on the presented image. The PC MRA demonstrates well the arterial feeders and to a lesser extent the AVF itself (which was better seen on individual axial sections, as opposed to the thick MIP presented). Lateral and frontal projections from DSA, with injection of the common carotid artery, are also presented. Venous drainage is via the transverse sinus and jugular bulb, the latter having a near complete occlusion at the exit from the skull base, with drainage of the AVF subsequently via the external jugular vein. No cerebellar cortical venous drainage was identified, classifying this dAVF as benign in type.

well as improved detection of very small lesions (**Fig. 6.14**). Small lesions will appear as discrete focal black dots on T2- and susceptibility weighted images. Mild heterogeneous contrast enhancement is common with all but the smallest lesions. MR is considered the imaging modality of choice for identification and long-term follow-up. On CT, large CCMs can be visualized and present as focal high-density lesions, commonly with associated calcification. On MR, an associated developmental venous anomaly (DVA) can be identified in 25%

of sporadic cases but is usually not seen in familial cases (**Fig. 6.15**).

CCMs are dynamic lesions and may spontaneously enlarge, regress, or form de novo. The risk of hemorrhage varies substantially between published studies and may be less than 1%, with many hemorrhages asymptomatic. An associated venous angioma is considered a risk factor for symptomatic hemorrhage. Asymptomatic lesions are not infrequently identified as an incidental finding on MR.

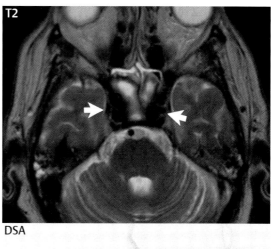

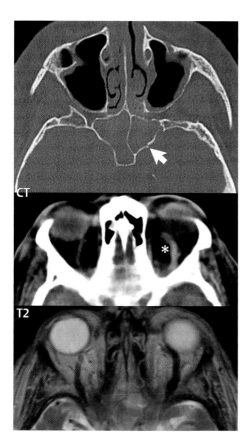

Fig. 6.13 Carotid cavernous fistula, traumatic. The images are all from the same patient. In Part 1, the axial CT reformatted with a bone algorithm reveals complete opacification of the sphenoid sinus by blood in this trauma patient, together with a fracture of the wall of the sinus on the left (*white arrow*). Fractures were also noted of the left occipital bone and petrous apex (not shown). The axial CT and MR through the orbits demonstrate an enlarged superior ophthalmic vein (*white asterisk*) on the left. This is seen as a flow void (dark) on the MR. In Part 2, prominent flow voids are seen within, together with engorgement of, both cavernous sinuses (*white arrows*). The frontal DSA projection from a left internal carotid artery injection reveals the shunt into the left cavernous sinus, with filling as well of the contralateral cavernous sinus and retrograde filling of the left superior ophthalmic vein (*black arrow*). There is prominent filling of the inferior petrosal sinuses bilaterally (*black asterisks*).

■ Developmental Venous Anomaly

The more descriptive term *developmental venous anomaly* (DVA) is now used in place of the older term venous angioma. In this entity, a stellate collection of peripheral veins (the "caput medusae") lying in white matter converge to a dilated central draining vein, an appearance well visualized on contrast-enhanced MR (**Fig. 6.16**). Although a very large DVA is illustrated, these occur in a spectrum of sizes, with the majority being small. Supratentorial DVAs typically drain toward the wall of the lateral ventricle, while infratentorial lesions drain into the sigmoid sinus. DVAs are usually solitary, are commonly visualized incidentally on contrast-enhanced MR, and are the most common asymptomatic vascular malformation of the brain. They are considered to be a normal variant of intraparenchymal medullary veins. It is important to note that these are, with rare exception, completely benign. DVAs can be confused by

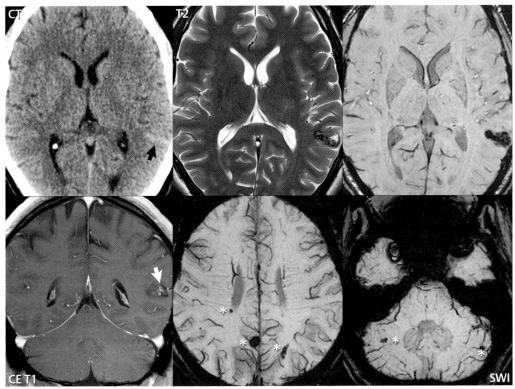

Fig. 6.14 Multiple cerebral cavernous malformations. The patient, a 43-year-old, presented with seizures. An ovoid lesion with increased density consistent with calcification on a precontrast CT (*black arrow*) and a reticulated "popcorn ball"–like appearance, with mixed signal intensity centrally and a complete hemosiderin rim on the T2-weighted scan, is identified in the superior temporal gyrus on the left. On the susceptibility weighted image (SWI; upper row on the right), due to greater T2* sensitivity (and thus impact of the susceptibility effect of the hemosiderin within the lesion), the lesion is uniformly low signal intensity. The lower two figures on the right are minimum intensity projection images from the SWI acquisition and demonstrate multiple additional smaller lesions (*asterisks*). Heterogeneous enhancement of the largest lesion (*white arrow*), a common finding, is seen on the coronal postcontrast T1-weighted scan.

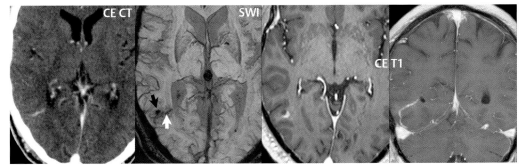

Fig. 6.15 Small cerebral cavernous malformation, with an associated developmental venous anomaly. On CT, only a small linear enhancing structure is noted. SWI reveals both a small cerebral cavernous malformation (*black arrow*) and the associated small draining vein (*white arrow*). On the axial postcontrast MR, the vein is noted coursing immediately posterior to the malformation. On the coronal postcontrast MR, the appearance is that of a solitary vein extending from the atrium of the lateral ventricle toward the transverse sinus. Close inspection of the high-resolution 3D postcontrast T1 weighted scan revealed multiple small tributary veins, the "caput," with drainage into the transverse sinus.

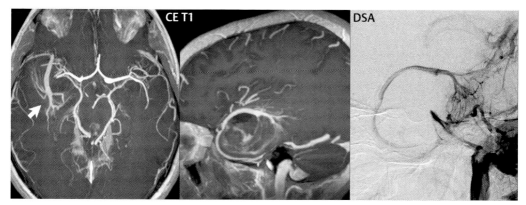

Fig. 6.16 Developmental venous anomaly (DVA). The patient presented with a large, acute temporal lobe hemorrhage. Imaging revealed a large associated DVA (*arrow*), which was confirmed on DSA. Axial and sagittal thin MIP projections from a contrast-enhanced T1-weighted 3D MP-RAGE exam are illustrated. A lateral projection from a delayed venous phase of the DSA exam is also presented for comparison. Note the dilated medullary veins, the caput or "Medusa head," draining via a single large anomalous vein, which courses anteriorly around the temporal lobe tip. The hemorrhage was presumed to be due to an associated cavernous malformation.

the novice with AVMs and, when associated with a CCM, can be erroneously identified as the source of symptoms. During surgery for resection of a CCM, if a DVA is present, it is critical that this be preserved. Resection of a DVA can cause a venous infarct. Autopsy series show DVAs in 3% of individuals, and in a large published series on MR, DVAs were identified in 1%.

■ Capillary Telangiectasia

Histologically a capillary telangiectasia is a cluster of enlarged, dilated capillaries interspersed with normal brain parenchyma. These are rare, clinically benign lesions, with the most common site being the pons (often centrally). MR imaging characteristics include a size < 1 cm, faint contrast enhancement, hypointensity on GRE and SWI, and in about half of cases, faint hyperintensity on FLAIR (**Fig. 6.17**). These are usually visualized incidentally, typically being quiescent without symptoms. CT is typically normal.

■ Vertebrobasilar Dolichoectasia

Vertebrobasilar dolichoectasia by definition involves both an increase in length ("dolicho") and diameter ("ectasia") of the involved vessels (**Fig. 6.18**, Parts 1 and 2). This entity is seen in the elderly with hypertension and atherosclerotic disease. In terms of the basilar artery, elongation results in the artery lying lateral to the clivus or dorsum sellae and/or terminating above the suprasellar cistern. A diameter

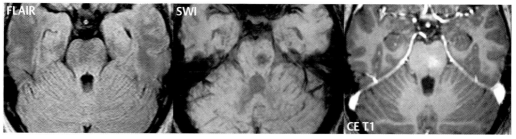

Fig. 6.17 Capillary telangiectasia. No abnormality is noted on FLAIR. A poorly defined lesion is seen in the left pons both on SWI and postcontrast, with moderate low signal intensity on the former and mild stippled enhancement on the latter. On adjacent sections (not shown), a tiny presumed draining vein was identified. **135**

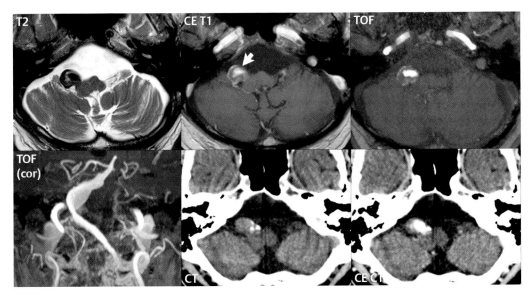

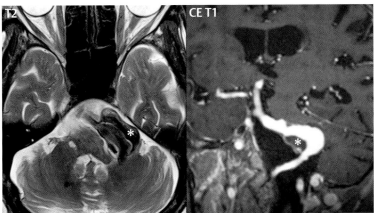

Fig. 6.18 Vertebrobasilar dolichoectasia, with clot (thrombus) within the ectatic basilar artery. In the exam from the first patient (Part 1), the basilar artery is large in diameter (ectatic) with mixed signal intensity therein on the axial T2-weighted scan. Postcontrast and TOF images confirm at this level a relatively normal caliber, patent lumen (with contrast enhancement, *arrow*), surrounded by clot. There is mass effect upon, and mild deformity of, the adjacent medulla. The coronal TOF MIP shows the elongation ("dolicho") of the basilar artery, which extends far to the right of midline, and then terminates very high. The patent portion of this markedly ectatic basilar artery is largest in its midsection. Similar findings are demonstrated at the level of the medulla on CT, with some associated vascular calcification. Findings in a second patient (Part 2) are similar, with axial T2-weighted and oblique coronal postcontrast T1-weighted scans revealing a markedly elongated, ectatic basilar artery with associated luminal clot (*asterisk*). It should be noted that the involvement of the vertebral arteries is variable, and often mild compared to that of the basilar artery.

> 4.5 mm on CT is considered to be ectatic. There can be marked (long-standing) deformity of the pons. Cranial nerve deficits can occur due to compression. In addition, intraluminal thrombus is not uncommon in symptomatic patients. However, vertebrobasilar dolichoectasia by itself is typically asymptomatic.

■ Venous Thrombosis

Dural venous sinus thrombosis has many etiologies and can be the result of infection, dehydration, trauma, neoplasia, oral contraceptives, pregnancy, or hematologic abnormalities. Patients present with signs of

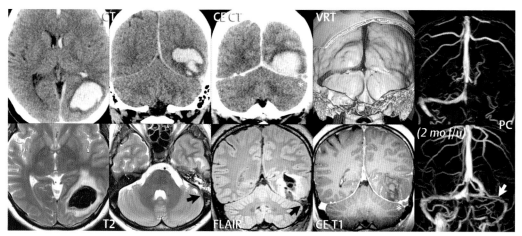

Fig. 6.19 Occlusion of the left transverse sinus by acute thrombus, with an accompanying occipital hematoma. On the CT at clinical presentation, a large acute occipital hematoma, with mild surrounding vasogenic edema and extension into the left lateral ventricle, is identified. A small acute subdural hematoma is also noted along the falx and left tentorium. There is abnormal hyperdensity in the left transverse sinus precontrast on the coronal reformat. Following contrast administration, there is a thin rim of enhancement circumferential to the sinus (*asterisk*), the empty delta sign (although this term is most commonly used in reference to the superior sagittal sinus). The VRT image shows nonfilling of the left transverse sinus. On the MR performed 2 days later, both the occipital hematoma and the clot within the transverse sinus (*black arrows*) are identified to be deoxyhemoglobin in composition, and thus have low signal intensity on T2-weighted scans. The equivalent on MR of the empty delta sign is also seen on the postcontrast coronal image, with nonenhancing thrombus centrally and a thin periphery of enhancement (*asterisk*). Phase contrast angiography (top row) at clinical presentation reveals a lack of flow in the left transverse and sigmoid sinuses, with partial recanalization (*arrow*) on the 2-month follow-up (lower row). The patient was on oral contraceptives and presented with headache, nausea, vomiting, and a right hemianopsia.

increased intracranial pressure, including specifically headache, nausea, papilledema, and lethargy. Venous infarction, specifically including hemorrhagic infarction, and parenchymal hemorrhage are known complications. Sinus thrombosis is treated medically with anticoagulants, with recanalization of the sinus in most instances long term (usually verified by follow-up MR). On precontrast CT, the sinus will be hyperdense, and on postcontrast CT, an "empty delta sign" will be seen, due to enhancement of venous collateral channels that surround the thrombosed sinus (**Fig. 6.19**).

On MR, the venous clot early on may be composed of deoxyhemoglobin, with low signal intensity therein on T2-weighted scans. This presentation is less common than that of a methemoglobin subacute clot; however, deoxyhemoglobin clots can be difficult to recognize and demand close inspection of images. Most visualized clots within the dural sinuses are methemoglobin in composition and easily recognized due to the high signal intensity within the clot on T1-weighted scans. Imaging of the dural sinus in two planes is recommended to avoid confusion with flow phenomena. Postcontrast on MR, there may be enhancement of small venous collaterals immediately surrounding the sinus. MR venography (MRV) is used to confirm the absence of flow within the sinus, most often with 2D TOF MRA techniques (which are sensitive to the slower flow within the dural sinuses). One caveat is the high signal intensity of methemoglobin on certain MRA sequences. Phase contrast MRA techniques can also be used and do not suffer from this potential pitfall. Although thrombosis of a dural venous sinus is most common, deep cerebral venous thrombosis and cortical vein thrombosis also occur.

■ Vascular Lesions (Neck)

CT angiography (CTA) and contrast-enhanced MR angiography (CE MRA) are commonly used today for evaluation of the carotid and vertebral arteries. The most frequent indication is atherosclerotic disease, with evaluation focused on the bifurcation of the common carotid artery (**Fig. 6.20**). Critical to this assessment is evaluation of stenosis, in the immediate vicinity of the bifurcation, involving either the distal common carotid artery or the proximal internal carotid artery. Stenosis of the latter is reported, preferably using cross-sectional area measurements, relative to (percentage wise) a more distal normal section of the internal carotid artery. Ulcerated plaques are well visualized by either modality and are important to recognize (**Fig 6.21**).

Atherosclerosis can cause cerebral ischemia by two mechanisms: hemodynamic compromise due to stenosis and embolization from an ulcerated plaque. Advances in medical therapy, specifically including antiplatelet therapy

and cholesterol-lowering medications, have had great impact on the treatment of both symptomatic and asymptomatic carotid stenosis. Asymptomatic stenosis usually follows a benign course, with medical management alone likely the best option. Carotid endarterectomy in selected high-risk patients with symptomatic stenosis can be beneficial.

CE MRA is typically performed with a field of view that extends from the aortic arch to the skull base, providing a broad assessment of atherosclerotic disease, with close inspection of all the major arteries visualized important due to the generalized nature of atherosclerotic disease. Time-resolved CE MRA enables assessment of the vascularity of mass lesions and provides information regarding arterial and venous flow. The latter is important for evaluation of vascular malformations and other vascular lesions such as subclavian steal syndrome.

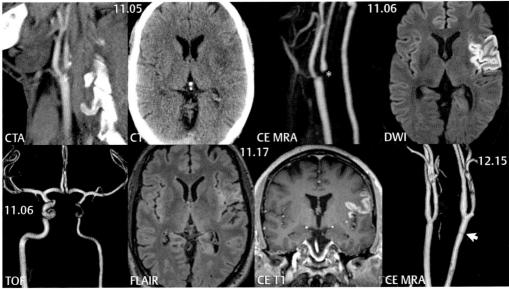

Fig. 6.20 Severe stenosis at the origin of the left internal carotid artery (ICA), with infarction in the left MCA territory. Both CTA and CE MRA reveal the severe stenosis (*asterisk*) at the origin of the ICA, with MRA also visualizing well the reduced caliber of the vessel subsequent to the carotid bulb. The initial axial CT, at the level of the frontal horns, demonstrates abnormal low density within a portion of the left MCA territory. There is restricted diffusion (confirmed on the ADC map) on DWI within the pre- and postcentral gyri, pars opercularis of the inferior frontal gyrus, and insula. Note the markedly reduced caliber of the distal left ICA on the AP thick MIP TOF MRA, indicative of a flow restriction more proximally. Eleven days later, little edema is visualized within the involved portion of the MCA territory on FLAIR (pseudo-normalization), with cortical enhancement seen on the coronal postcontrast T1-weighted scan, reflecting blood-brain barrier disruption now present within this subacute infarct. A month later, a carotid endarterectomy was performed. The VRT image displays the now widely patent origin of the left ICA, with the proximal edge of the endarterectomy (*arrow*) also visible.

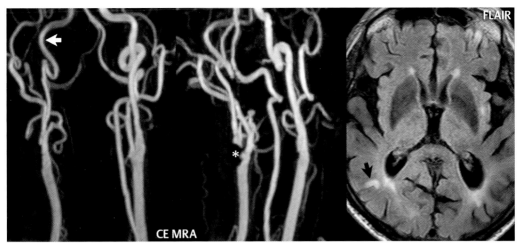

Fig. 6.21 Symptomatic high-grade stenosis at the origin of the right internal carotid artery. This 83-year-old hypertensive man presented clinically with signs of an MCA infarct. Two views from an MIP rotation of the CE MRA study of the carotid bifurcations reveal a smaller diameter and lower signal intensity distal right internal carotid artery (*white arrow*), findings consistent with a more proximal symptomatic stenosis. A very high-grade stenosis, with nonvisualization of a short segment of the proximal internal carotid artery, is visualized on the right, together with a small, ulcerated plaque (*asterisk*). Atherosclerotic narrowing and carotid plaque ulceration (the latter independent of the degree of stenosis) are well-recognized causes of cerebral infarction. On the axial FLAIR scan, a small cortical infarct with abnormal high signal intensity (*black arrow*) is identified within the middle temporal gyrus. The lesion also demonstrated restricted diffusion (image not shown).

Dissection of the internal carotid artery can be spontaneous, posttraumatic, or due to an underlying predisposing arteriopathy (for example, fibromuscular dysplasia, Marfan, or Ehlers-Danlos). A history of minor trauma is present in nearly half of cases, with chiropractic manipulation a common cause. In terms of pathogenesis, blood enters the wall of the artery through an intimal tear, forming an intramural hematoma. The typical clinical presentation is that of unilateral neck pain, often with facial pain and headache. Horner's syndrome is common, featuring a constricted pupil, ptosis, and anhydrosis. The initial clinical presentation may be followed by ischemic symptoms in hours or days due to thromboembolism. Therapy is antithrombotic, with aspirin or anticoagulation.

CTA and CE MRA both depict well the luminal narrowing in dissection of the internal carotid artery, together with (if present) focal aneurysmal dilatation. The latter occurs in 30%, typically immediately prior to the internal carotid artery entering the carotid canal at the skull base. The dissection itself can extend for a variable length, often originating a few centimeters distal to the carotid bulb. The intramural hematoma is usually well delineated on precontrast axial T1-weighted MR scans with fat saturation, on which the methemoglobin in the hematoma will be seen as a hyperintense crescent adjacent to the residual patent lumen. Although typical, the hematoma need not be hyperintense on T1-weighted scans; it can be isointense in the very early stages and is usually isointense when chronic (**Fig. 6.22**). Both CTA and CE MRA perform less well for the diagnosis of vertebral artery dissection.

Venous thrombosis, in particular that of the internal jugular vein, has many etiologies, including drug abuse, central venous catheterization, compression by benign or malignant disease, hypercoagulable states, and infection. The thrombosed vein is typically enlarged in the acute and subacute time frame, with peripheral enhancement of the vessel wall and surrounding inflammation. Collateral venous channels may develop with chronic thrombosis, with the (occluded) internal jugular vein itself small.

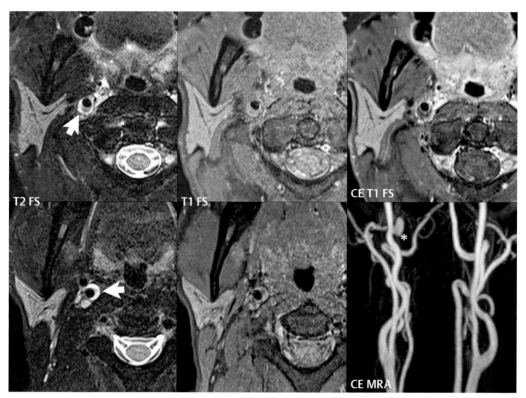

Fig. 6.22 Acute internal carotid artery dissection. The patient presented with Horner's syndrome. An intramural hematoma (fluid collection, *arrows*) is best seen on the T2-weighted scans with fat saturation (two axial levels are illustrated). There is only a mild reduction in the caliber of the involved carotid artery. Although a dissection in many instances is high signal intensity on a T1-weighted scan, reflecting methemoglobin, this need not be the case (as in the current example). In such instances, a postcontrast T1-weighted image with fat saturation may improve visualization of the lesion, due to mild enhancement of adjacent tissues and the vessel wall. On the CE MRA, a pseudoaneurysm (*asterisk*) is also noted, located near the skull base and distal to the axial images presented. A reduction in caliber of the internal carotid artery is not evident on the MIP of the CE MRA study, other than at the location of the pseudoaneurysm.

Index

Page numbers followed by f indicate figures.

1.5 T, 1, 3–8, 10–15, 19–20, 44, 4f, 6–8f, 10–13f, 17f, 19f
2D time of flight, 85, 117, 137
3 T, 1–20, 22, 40, 42, 44, 46, 71, 78, 96, 108–110, 121, 126, 2f, 4f, 6–8f, 10–13f, 17f, 19f
3D time of flight, 7–9, 37, 117, 8–9f, 61f, 97f
3D TOF. See 3D time of flight

A
Abnormal contrast enhancement, infarct, 59, 59f
ACA infarct, 63, 68f
ACA. See Anterior cerebral artery
ACOM. See Anterior communicating artery
Acute hypertensive encephalopathy, 92
Acute infarct, 48, 52, 76, 25f, 32f, 64f, 66f, 70f, 73f, 81–84f, 88–89f, 119f
Acute MCA occlusion, 51f, 54f
ADC. See Apparent diffusion coefficient
AICA. See Anterior inferior cerebellar artery
Anatomic variant, 37, 75, 107
Aneurysm, 7, 29, 34, 40, 95–121, 123–125, 129, 8f
  ACOM, 102f, 108f, 114–115f
  anterior cerebral, 105, 107, 109f
  anterior choroidal, 100f, 107f
  basilar artery, 96f
  basilar tip, 110f
  carotid cave, 104f
  carotid terminus, 97f
  cavernous carotid (cavernous ICA), 103, 95f, 103f
  comparison of surgery and endovascular treatment, 101, 117
  dolichoectatic aneurysm, 118
  endovascular treatment, 99–101, 117
  flow diversion, 101
  fusiform aneurysm, 118
  giant aneurysms, 117–118, 120f
  hydrocephalus, 116, 114f
  infectious aneurysms (embolic, mycotic), 117, 118f
  MCA, 107, 8f, 96f, 109f, 112f
  occlusion (coiling), 99–102, 97f, 99–102f, 105–106f, 108f, 110f, 116f
  ophthalmic artery, 98f, 105f
  paraclinoid ICA, 103–104
  partially thrombosed, 120f
  PCOM, 101f, 106f, 116f
  pericallosal, 109f
  PICA, 111f
  posterior circulation, 107, 110
  recanalization, 102f
  recurrent, 99f
  ruptured, 114–116f
  subarachnoid hemorrhage, 110–111, 116–117
  supraclinoid, 104–105
  surgical treatment, 98–99, 117
  traumatic aneurysm, 118
  treatment, 98–102, 117
  vasospasm, 101, 116–117
Anterior cerebral artery (ACA), 4, 30–32, 34, 48, 54, 63–64, 70, 72, 95, 105, 107, 115, 121, 123, 68f, 90–91f, 121f, 125f
Anterior choroidal artery, 30, 100, 104, 107, 30f
Anterior communicating artery (ACOM), 30, 34, 95, 105, 107, 68f, 102f, 108f, 114–115f
Anterior inferior cerebellar artery (AICA), 32, 63–64, 33f, 69f, 124f
Anterior spinal artery, 32, 33f
Apparent diffusion coefficient (ADC), 4, 21, 52, 57–59, 69, 85, 88, 50–51f, 71f, 73f, 77–78f, 84f, 88f, 89f, 94f, 138f
Arachnoid granulations, 35, 38
Arterial spin labeling (ASL), 16, 20f
Arterial territory infarct, 63
Arterial territory, 63–64
Arteriovenous fistula (AVF), 110–111, 125–126, 129, 130–132f
Arteriovenous malformation (AVM), 97, 110–111, 121–129, 135, 121–129f
ASL. See arterial spin labeling
Atherosclerosis, 47–48, 138, 85f
Atrophy, 52, 60–62, 93, 61f, 67f, 125f
AVF. See Arteriovenous fistula
AVM. See Arteriovenous malformation

B
b value, 58
Basilar artery, 5, 32–34, 56, 63 64, 96, 110, 135–136
Behçet's disease, 93
BLADE, 14–15, 16f
Blood product degradation. See deoxyhemo-globin; hemosiderin; methemoglobin
Brain death, 54
Brain screening, 5
Brainstem infarct, 75–76
Brainstem, 27, 29, 31–33, 52–53, 63, 72, 75–77, 93, 118
Broca's area, 27, 48, 82f
Bulk susceptibility, 5, 8, 13f

C

CADASIL, 93
Capillary telangiectasia, 135, 135f
Caput medusae, 133, 134–135f
Carbon monoxide poisoning, 92
Carotid artery, 6, 9, 26, 29–31, 33–34, 47–48,
    61, 63, 68, 70, 72, 90–91, 95, 97, 100,
    104, 107, 117–118, 130, 132–133,
    138–140, 30–31f
Carotid cavernous fistula, 133f
Caudate head, 2, 25, 30, 63, 32f
Caudate nucleus, 31, 48, 63, 64f
Cavernous malformation, 19, 130, 134f
CBF. See Cerebral blood flow
CBV. See Cerebral blood volume
CE MRA, 137–139, 89f, 138–140f,
CE TOF MRA, 132f
Cerebellum, 27–29, 31–32, 44, 63–64, 72, 94
Cerebral blood flow (CBF), 16, 19, 23, 49,
    51–52, 117, 24f, 26f, 53f
Cerebral blood volume (CBV), 19, 23, 51, 21f,
    23f, 51f, 54–55f, 58f, 68f
Cerebral edema, 14, 117
Cerebral proliferative angiopathy, 125
Chronic infarct, 55–56, 58–61, 60–61f
Clot, 25, 40, 43, 48, 72, 137, 40–41f, 86–87f,
    120f, 136–137f
CNR, 5, 7–8, 23
Contrast enhancement, 5, 7, 54–55, 59–60,
    75, 121–122, 132, 135, 7f, 106f, 122f,
    136f
Contrast media, 5, 23
Contrast-enhanced, 117, 133, 137, 86f, 95f,
    97f, 110–111f, 123f, 129f, 131–132f,
    135f
Contusion, 93, 94f
Corticospinal tract, 29, 61, 62f
CT angiography (CTA), 20, 23–24, 26, 49, 51,
    97–98, 111, 116–117, 122, 129, 137, 139,
    26f, 47f, 51f, 68–69f, 89–91f, 95f, 112f,
    114–116f, 119–120f, 123–124f, 127f,
    131f, 138f
CTA. See CT angiography
Cystic change, 60, 93, 60f
Cystic encephalomalacia, 60, 55f, 60f, 69f
Cytotoxic edema, 12, 14, 49, 52–53, 58, 2f,
    15f, 65–66f, 71–73f, 77f, 89f

D

DAI. See Diffuse axonal injury
dAVF. See Dural arteriovenous fistula
Deep venous system, 36–37, 37f
Demyelination, 85, 91, 93
Dense MCA sign, 50, 23f, 51f
Deoxyhemoglobin, 16, 40, 57–58, 137, 17f,
    40f, 42f, 44f, 51–52f, 82f, 87f, 94f,
    137f
Detector design, CT, 23–24
Developmental venous anomaly (DVA),
    132–133, 135f

Diffuse axonal injury (DAI), 93, 94f
Diffusion-weighted imaging (DWI), 5, 8, 14,
    16, 20, 24, 49, 53, 57–59, 75, 4f, 11–15f,
    22f, 50–51f, 53–56f, 59–60f, 62–66f,
    68–74f, 77–78f, 79–84f, 86–89f, 94f,
    100f, 119f, 138f
Digital subtraction angiography (DSA), 21, 25,
    43, 53, 111, 35f, 54–56f, 60f, 68f, 70f, 91f,
    96–97f, 99–108f, 110f, 114–116f, 120f,
    122–133f, 135f
Dilated perivascular space, 37, 75, 75f
Direct carotid-cavernous fistula (CCF), 129–130
Dissection, 49, 76, 139, 47f, 140f
DSA. See Digital subtraction angiography
Dual energy CT, 20–21, 25
Dural arteriovenous fistula (dAVF), 125–126,
    129, 130–132f
DVA. See Developmental venous anomaly
DWI. See Diffusion-weighted imaging
Dynamic susceptibility contrast, 16

E

Early subacute infarct, 55, 2f, 10f, 17f
Echo planar imaging, 8
Emboli, 48, 71–72, 117, 73f
Embolic infarct, 71–72
Encephalomalacia, 60, 63, 93, 55f, 60f, 69f
Extension (of an infarct), 88, 89f
External carotid artery, 34, 90, 130, 130f, 132f

F

Falx cerebri, 34
Fat saturation, 139, 140f
Field strength, 1–8, 16, 18, 40, 44, 11f, 17f
FLAIR, 3, 5, 14–15, 41–42, 49, 52–53, 56,
    59–61, 85, 90, 92–93, 135, 14–16f, 18f,
    28f, 42f, 44–45f, 53f, 55–56f, 60–62f, 65f,
    67f, 69–71f, 73f, 77–78f, 80f, 84–86f, 92f,
    94f, 97f, 113f, 135f, 138–139f
Flow diversion, 101–102
Fogging, 56
Fracture, 118, 129, 45f, 94f, 113f, 133f
Frontal lobe, 27, 64, 76, 79, 45f, 79f, 86f, 98f,
    114f

G

Gadolinium, 5–6, 16, 18, 7f
Gliosis, 4, 56, 60–61, 75, 88, 93, 122, 28f, 45f,
    55f, 60–62f, 67f, 69f, 71f, 78f, 125f
Gradient echo, 3, 5–7, 44, 131, 6f, 12f, 17f,
    19f, 97f, 110f, 121f, 129f
GRE, 5–6, 57, 59, 131, 135, 6f, 17f, 42f,
    44–45f, 75f, 87f, 103f, 106f, 122f, 126f
Gyral localization, 76, 79, 83

H

HASTE, 14–15, 15f
Hematoma, 40–41, 49, 55, 75, 125, 139, 18f,
    39–41f, 86f, 119f, 126f, 127f, 131f, 137f,
    140f

Hemorrhage, 12, 15–16, 21, 39–44, 49, 55–58, 85, 93, 95–97, 99, 103–105, 107, 110–111, 116–117, 121–126, 129, 131–132, 135, 137, 17f, 25f, 39f, 39–46f, 51–52f, 54f, 57f, 61f, 82f, 86–87f, 94f, 113–116f, 119f, 123f, 126–127f, 131f, 137f
    acute hypertensive, 39f, 92f
    parenchymal, 39–41, 39–41f, 45f, 51–52f, 82f, 86–87f, 94f, 119f, 123f, 126–127f, 131f, 137f
    subarachnoid, 41–43, 96–97, 110–111, 43–45f, 113–116f
    temporal progression, 40, 40f, 41f
    ventricular, 43, 46f, 126f
Hemorrhagic transformation, 55, 57f
Hemosiderin cleft, 41, 40f
Hemosiderin, 15–16, 40–41, 44, 57–58, 75, 122, 131, 19f, 40–42f, 45–46f, 52f, 61f, 75f, 87f, 118f, 123f, 134f
Herniation, 25f
Homunculus, 27, 76
Hydrocephalus, 90, 116, 126, 46f, 114f, 116f
Hyperacute hemorrhage, 40
Hypertensive encephalopathy, 92, 92f
Hypertensive hemorrhage, 40, 39f
Hypotension, 55, 71, 59f, 72f

I
Imaging technique, 1–2, 53, 12f, 71f, 97f
Increased speed, CT, 24
Indirect carotid-cavernous fistula (CCF), 129–130
Infarction, 14, 23, 31, 47–48, 50, 59, 63–64, 68, 71–72, 75–76, 79, 83, 85, 88, 90, 93, 125, 137, 4f, 24f, 26f, 32f, 45f, 52f, 61f, 63–75f, 77–84f, 86–90f, 138–139f
Infection, 117, 136, 139
Inflammation, 95, 139, 118f
Insula, 27, 31, 63, 79, 47f, 51f, 83f, 138f
Insular cortex, 27, 50
Iron, 93
Iterative reconstruction, CT, 20–21

K
k-space, 9, 12–13, 15–16
kVp, 20, 22–24

L
Lacunar infarct, 2, 14, 37, 48, 52–53, 55, 59, 72, 75, 71f, 73f
Lenticulostriate artery (arteries), 30–31, 37, 63, 90, 31–32f, 64f, 91f
Lentiform nucleus, 37, 10f, 23f, 32f, 54f
Low peak kilovoltage, 22–23

M
Magnetic resonance angiography (MRA), 7–8, 37, 90, 97, 98, 116–118, 122, 137–139, 8–9f, 21f, 35f, 47f, 55–56f, 61f, 70f, 89f, 91f, 95–98f, 101–111f, 116f, 118f, 121–123f, 125–128f, 130f, 132f, 138–140f
Magnetic resonance venography (MRV), 137
Magnetic susceptibility, 8, 18, 40, 57, 75f, 105f
MCA. See Middle cerebral artery
Mean transit time (MTT), 16, 19, 23, 51–52, 55, 21f, 24f, 51f, 55f
Medulla, 29, 31, 61, 63, 76, 78, 69f, 136f
Medullary infarct, 76, 11f, 22f, 69f, 78f
Meningitis, 41, 90–91, 117
Metal artifact, 8, 21, 98f
Metastatic disease, 7, 92
Methemoglobin, 5, 15, 40–41, 43, 56–58, 137, 139, 17–18f, 39–40f, 52f, 87f, 140f
Middle cerebral artery (MCA), 5, 15, 31, 48–50, 63–64, 95, 105, 107, 117, 121, 123, 2f, 8f, 10f, 21f, 23f, 25–26f, 31–32f, 35f, 47f, 51–57f, 60–63f, 68f, 70f, 72f, 83–84f, 89–91f, 96–97f, 99f, 109f, 112f, 121f, 125f, 127f, 138–139f
MIP, 8–9f, 77f, 86–87f, 91f, 97–98f, 101–103f, 105–106f, 108–112f, 116f, 122f, 126f, 128–132f, 135–136f, 138–140f
Mitochondrial Encephalomyopathy with Lactic Acidosis and Stroke-Like Episodes (MELAS), 93
Motion artifact, 2–3, 5, 14–15, 15–16f
Motion, 2–3, 5, 8–9, 12, 14–15, 15–16f, 82f
Motor hand area, 76, 80f
Moyamoya, 90, 20f, 91f
MP-RAGE, 6–7, 78f, 97f, 107f, 135f
MRA. See Magnetic resonance angiography
MRV. See Magnetic resonance venography
MS. See Multiple sclerosis
MTT. See Mean transit time
Multiple sclerosis (MS), 76, 85, 90

N
Normal anatomy, 27–38, 30–31f, 33f, 36f, 37f
Normal variant, 30, 34, 133, 75f

O
Obstructive hydrocephalus, 46f, 114f, 116f
Occipital lobe, 27, 31, 60, 63, 79, 83, 59f, 65f, 113f, 84f, 89f
Orbit, 27, 36, 133f
Osmotic demyelination, 93
Oxyhemoglobin, 40

P
Paradigm, 100
Parenchymal hemorrhage, 39–41, 39–41f, 45f, 51–52f, 82f, 86–87f, 94f, 119f, 123f, 126–127f, 131f, 137f
Parietal lobe, 27, 63, 76, 79, 55f, 65f, 126f

PC. See Phase contrast
PCA. See Posterior cerebral artery
PCOM. See Posterior communicating artery
pCT. See Perfusion CT
Perfusion CT (pCT), 23, 50–52, 23f
Perfusion imaging, 16, 18–20, 23, 84f
Perfusion, 1, 16, 20, 23–24, 49–53, 55, 71,
    117, 20–21f, 23–24f, 26f, 53f, 55f, 68f, 84f
Perivascular space, 37–38, 75, 75f
Petechial hemorrhage, 16, 49, 55, 17f, 57f
Petrous apex, 36, 12–13f
Phase contrast (PC), 37, 132, 86f, 121f, 127f,
    129f, 132f
PICA. See Posterior inferior cerebellar artery
Pipeline, 100, 102
Pons, 29, 32, 40, 48, 61, 75–76, 93, 110,
    135–136, 12f, 62f, 77f, 135f
Pontine infarct, 76, 12f, 16f, 77f
Postcentral gyrus, 27, 29, 61, 76, 15f, 51–52f,
    61f, 73f, 81f, 121f, 138f
Posterior cerebral artery (PCA), 5, 31, 34,
    48, 59–60, 63–64, 95, 110, 10f, 33f,
    58f, 65–67f, 70f, 72f, 75f, 89–90f, 106f,
    124–125f, 128f
Posterior communicating artery (PCOM),
    29–31, 34, 95–96, 103–105, 107, 30f, 68f,
    99f, 101f, 106f, 116f, 128f
Posterior inferior cerebellar artery (PICA),
    31–32, 63–64, 76, 110, 33f, 69f, 90f,
    111f, 124f
Precentral gyrus, 27, 48, 76, 79, 81, 53f, 73f,
    80–81f
Primary motor cortex, 27, 48, 61, 76
Primary somatosensory cortex, 27, 29, 76, 81f
Putamen, 30–31, 40, 48, 63, 32f, 39f, 64f

R
Radiation dose reduction, CT, 24
Radiation dose, CT, 1, 20, 22–24, 123
Radiation injury, 91
Radiation therapy, 91
Radiation white matter changes, 92
Readout-segmented, 3, 5, 8, 20, 13f
rs-EPI, 9, 12, 13f, 22f

S
SCA. See Superior cerebellar artery
Sickle cell disease, 49, 88
Simultaneous multislice, 1, 20, 22f
Sinus thrombosis, 85, 111, 136–137, 137f
Sinusitis, 68f
Skull (skull base), 29, 118, 129, 138–139,
    132f, 140f
Slice thickness, 1, 3–6, 2f, 4f, 10–12f, 17f, 19f, 42f
Small vessel ischemic disease, 83, 85
SNR, 1–3, 5, 7–8, 16, 20, 23, 4f, 8f, 13f, 16–17f,
    19–20f
SPACE, 7
Spatial resolution, 1–3, 6–9, 20, 24, 38, 2f, 8f,
    10–11f

ss-EPI, 8–9, 12, 13f, 22f
Stenosis, 51, 71, 90, 124, 126, 129, 138, 35f,
    55–56f, 60–61f, 70f, 138–139f
Subacute hemorrhage, 40–41, 137
Subacute infarct, 54–60, 75, 2f, 4f, 10–13f,
    17f, 47f, 65f, 138f
Subarachnoid hemorrhage, 40–44, 96–97,
    103–105, 107, 110–111, 117, 43–45f,
    113–116f
Subdural hematoma, 125, 18f, 137f
Superficial siderosis, 44
Superior cerebellar artery (SCA), 32, 64, 33f,
    96f, 123f
Surgery, 88, 97–99, 101, 104–105, 107,
    116–117, 123–124, 135, 58–59f, 88f, 90f,
    98f, 107f
Susceptibility artifact, 5, 8–9, 12–13f
Susceptibility-weighted imaging (SWI), 57,
    131, 41–42f, 45–46f, 87f, 94f, 134f
SWI. See Susceptibility-weighted imaging
Systemic lupus erythematosus, 88

T
T2*, 15–16, 18, 40, 42–44, 57, 59, 17f, 19f,
    42f, 44–45f, 51f, 75f, 82f, 87f, 134f
Temporal bone, 24, 35–36, 94f
Temporal evolution, hemorrhage, 40–41f
Temporal evolution, infarction, 75, 59–60f,
    67f, 69f, 71f
Temporal lobe, 27, 31, 36–37, 63, 79, 45f, 60f,
    63f, 65–67f, 135f
Thalamic infarct, 13f, 65f, 75f
Thalamus, 30–31, 36, 40, 63, 72, 75, 85, 14f,
    65f, 67f, 75f, 87f
Thrombectomy, 49, 53–54, 54f, 68f
Thrombolysis, 49, 53, 25f, 50–53f
Thrombus, 35, 85, 117–118, 136, 51f, 68f,
    136–137f
Time of flight (TOF), 7–8, 37, 85, 97, 117, 122,
    137, 8–9f, 21f, 35f, 47f, 55–56f, 61f, 67f,
    70f, 91f, 95–98f, 101–111f, 116f, 118f,
    121–130f, 132f, 136f, 138f
Time to peak (TTP), 23f, 53–54f
TOF. See Time of flight
Trauma, 47, 93, 111, 118, 129, 136, 139, 45f,
    94f, 98f, 113f, 133f
TTP. See Time to peak
Tuberculosis, 90–91

U
Unenhanced CT, 122, 23f, 68f, 84f, 95f, 99f,
    113f, 119f, 124f, 126f

V
Vasculitis, 47, 53–54, 88, 93, 111, 56f
Vasogenic edema, 5, 14, 49, 52, 54–58, 88,
    91–93, 122, 4f, 15f, 39f, 40–41f, 47f,
    50–52f, 59f, 65–67f, 71f, 77–78f, 80f, 82f,
    84f, 86f, 94f, 118–119f, 126–127f, 131f
Vein of Galen, 34, 37, 36–37f

Venous angioma, see Developmental venous anomaly
Venous infarct, 85, 88, 125, 135, 137, 86f, 87f
Venous sinus thrombosis, 136–137, 137f
Venous sinus, 125–126, 136–137
Venous system, 34–37, 36–37f
Venous thrombosis, 85, 136–137, 139, 87f
Ventricles, 43, 85, 46f, 60f, 72f, 116f
Vertebral artery, 31–32, 34, 63, 76, 110, 138–139, 33f, 69f, 111f, 122f, 136f
Vertebrobasilar dolichoectasia, 118, 135–136, 136f
Virchow-Robin space, 37
Visual field defect, 59f, 84f

Volume rendering technique (VRT), 24, 91f, 95–98f, 101–102f, 105–107f, 109–111f, 114–115f, 120f, 137–138f
VRT. See Volume rendering technique

W
Wallerian degeneration, 61, 62f
Watershed infarct, 64, 28f, 60f, 70–71f
Watershed territory, 2f, 25f, 32f, 70f, 89–90f
Watershed, 64, 71–72, 88, 2f, 10f, 25f, 32f, 59–60f, 63f, 70–72f, 83f, 89–90f
Wernicke's area, 27, 48